Rewriting
Nursing History

 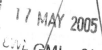

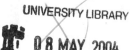
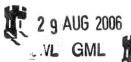

© 1980 Celia Davies   Chapter Three, Katherine Williams
Croom Helm Ltd, 2–10 St John's Road, London SW11

British Library Cataloguing in Publication Data

Rewriting nursing history
    1. Nursing – Great Britain –
    History
    I. Davies, Celia
    610.73'0941   RT11

    ISBN 0-85664-956-2
    ISBN 0-85664-992-9 Pbk

First published in the USA 1980 by

BARNES & NOBLE BOOKS
81 ADAMS DRIVE
TOTOWA, New Jersey, 07512

ISBN 0-389-20153-7

Typeset in Great Britain by
Pintail Studios Ltd, Ringwood, Hampshire

Printed in Great Britain

CONTENTS

"FIFTY

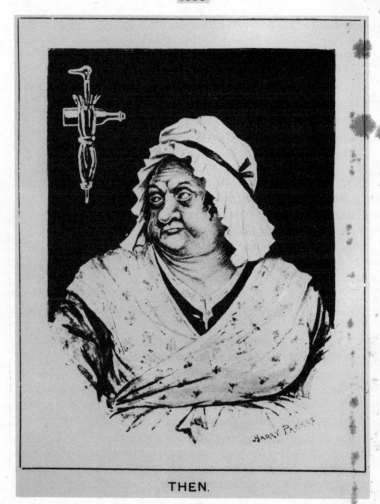

THEN.

Supplement to the "NURSING

(The "Nursing Record" is Published every Thursday, Price 2d.

Proprietors :

YEARS."

1888.

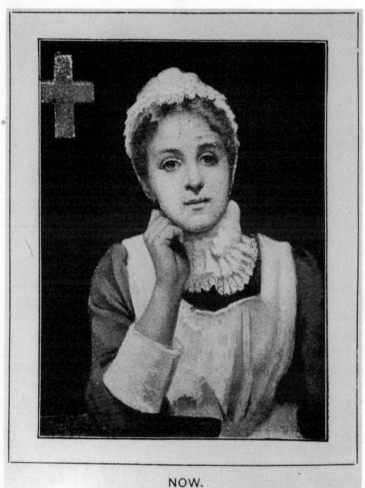

NOW.

RECORD," December 20, 1888.

Office, Dorset Works, Salisbury Square, Fleet Street, London.)

SAMPSON LOW, MARSTON, SEARLE AND RIVINGTON (Limited).

PREFACE

This collection of essays has come about as a result of certain personal experiences. Starting in 1977 on what was for me a new research project on nursing history, I was struck by the interest shown by members of the nursing profession in new accounts of their history. This came not only from tutors wanting new material to teach but from individuals who were interested in the history of nurses in their own locality, what source materials were there, how they might be saved and how they might be studied. It is a matter of regret to me that I have not, in the end, been able to include a local history in this collection.

Even more surprising and pleasant was the discovery that I was not alone in working in this field. I met, at various times, upwards of a dozen others with whom I was able to compare notes and exchange ideas. There were considerable divergences in what we severally were trying to achieve but we had in common a dissatisfaction with much existing nursing history and a feeling that new departures, based on developments in historical writing and in sociology, were in the air. My colleagues shared my view that, if these developments were more widely known, a process of 'rewriting nursing history' could begin. We were all working towards something which was more intellectually satisfying and at the same time more relevant to practising nurses too.

Not all of these people I met in the course of my work have become contributors to this volume. Some had other commitments already when the book was suggested and some are colleagues who emerged at a late stage of the production of the book. Had resources permitted, it would have been stimulating deliberately to bring together this little band of researchers for a fuller exchange of ideas. But I doubt that it would have produced a more integrated volume, or that any of them would have wanted to integrate their work very closely. For our common commitment is to developing diverse approaches and questioning an orthodox history of nursing.

I hope that the audience for this book will in large measure be nurses themselves. Those taking advanced courses with a history component will not be able to use this as 'the textbook'; I hope they will be able to use it as a collateral reading and one which helps them to develop a critical perspective towards the established texts. Beyond this, I would hope both to interest individual nurses and make them more critical of history, and to interest some historians and stimulate them also to enter, along with others, into this field. Above all, we need more work and more debate.

I would like to extend my thanks to the many nurses, historians and sociologists who have offered help and encouragement with this work on nursing history. I am especially grateful to my nurse colleagues in the Medical Sociology Group at the University of Warwick, whose enthusiasm provided a stimulus, and to Margaret Stacey who made this 'Warwick connection' possible. I would also extend especial thanks to Brenda Waller for her good humour and hard work in typing drafts and redrafts of the various chapters and to Penny Buckle for her additional last-minute help.

Celia Davies

1 INTRODUCTION: THE CONTEMPORARY CHALLENGE IN NURSING HISTORY

Celia Davies

There is a conventional form of writing nursing history which will be familiar to many readers of this volume. It involves broad-brush history, covering centuries rather than decades. It offers a connected, chronological narrative of events at a national and sometimes international level. Its focus is particularly upon individuals, leaders in the field, exceptional people who struggle against the odds and win. And it is evaluative, indeed largely congratulatory, in so far as it sees the history of nursing as an advance, as progress out of the dark ages to the present, modern times. The contributors to this volume share a scepticism about the value of this kind of history; singly and collectively they offer a challenge to each of the features listed above. To set the scene, then, for what follows, a brief discussion of these aspects of conventional history and the emerging challenge to them is in order.

Our frontispiece captures the view of 'history as progress' in a vivid pictorial form. Drawn from the journal, the *Nursing Record*, it served in the 1880s as a special pictorial supplement on nursing history. The old, ugly, wrinkled, fat character looks away from us, a sure sign of a shifty and unreliable person. She is bleary-eyed and the cause of her obvious preoccupation is something on which one would hesitate to enquire. The attractive, pure and unsullied-looking young woman, the new and modern nurse, holds our gaze in a calm and coolly attentive way. There is a cross behind her, not a bottle and a gamp.[1] What a transformation, what a clear advance in fifty years. Could anyone deny it?

There is nothing peculiar to nursing history in adopting this stance on progress. It has been pointed out, for example, that histories of professions are often written from within and written with a special professional purpose, namely to 'give the neophyte an everlasting faith in his profession'. This observation comes from a quite different field of activity.[2] We should note too that there are a great number of official histories (of hospitals, of associations, etc.) which are constrained to be evaluative and to give us evaluations which, by and large, are positive ones. But the assumption of history as advance goes much deeper than this. Butterfield, writing in the 1930s, was one of the first to point to the tendency to emphasise progress in history, to produce a story 'which is the ratification if not the glorification of the present'.[3] He termed this the Whig interpretation of history. E. P. Thompson has made a similar point, referring scathingly to a 'Pilgrim's Progress' view of history, which in his view is an 'orthodoxy in which the present is ransacked for forerunners, pioneers . . .'[4]

One of the important features which renders this position unacceptable to many scholars, and certainly to the contributors to this volume, is the theory of social change which underlies it. Implicit in what is written is a liberal–democratic view of change; it assumes that there is a group (or sometimes only a few individuals) with progressive and humanitarian ideas, it assumes that these ideas will find a forum of expression and it assumes that, being more just, these ideas will eventually win out against the opposition of vested interests. Other theoretical positions start from different perspectives – assuming that ruling ideas are much more hegemonic and less easily overthrown, denying that the political system is so open, seeing certain groups as consistently discriminated against, arguing that reforms are not necessarily progressive but are double-edged, always in part at least reflecting the views of the most powerful.

Of course, if these basic theoretical commitments endorsing specific views about the nature of society and the manner of social change were always quite explicitly stated, the quarrel with the liberal–democratic position would be less intense. It would be a matter of developing competing perspectives, exposing them to the test, asking why we should accept one particular account of history rather than another. As it is, the position is rather different. The liberal–democratic view is entrenched as conventional wisdom, it is so taken for granted that we neither see it nor discuss it and our critical faculties are blunted. The challenge, then, as seen by the various writers in this volume, is to start from the assumption that there is always a theoretical position, always a set of questions guiding the analysis. This is why a number of them see fit to start with a preamble on their own theoretical position, a position in most cases developed out of a critique of conventional history.

Conventional history does not appear as a history governed by theory; it appears as a narrative of events, which sets out historical facts. But 'facts' do not spring out of history unbidden. They emerge as salient and significant to particular people with particular questions in view. Other questions could well produce other facts and it is just as vital to examine the questions asked as to examine the answers given. Historians have often in the past been content to give their readers a narrative account which is coherent and connected. They have left to one side issues of theory and methods. What questions puzzled them? What sources did they consult? What did they discard? What did they count as relevant – and why? Such questions do not readily spring to mind when the reader is presented with a plausible account. The material set out is, by definition, consistent with the historian's interpretation. But differing questions might have led to different sources, and further plausible accounts. The more reflective kind of history exemplified in these essays is undoubtedly less easy to read, for it has a structure more complex than a chronological narrative. On the other hand, it provides, as the conventional narrative so rarely does, a basis for comparison, criticism and reflection.

When alternative theories are used, other features of conventional history come under question too, for theory and method are inter-related. The broad-brush overview is not necessarily the best way to tackle history when it is seen as something other than a series of advances. A much more detailed inquiry at particular moments selected for their comparability, for instance, might be called for; and it might become necessary to take a much shorter period and to concentrate as much on what was happening outside nursing as within it. The selection of sources might well be different also. A striking development in social history of late has been oral history – the growing concern with what is called 'history from below', the views and experiences of the rank and file. These views can sometimes only be captured through the reminiscences of participants, and are subject to all the difficulties and distortions which the retrospective interview method brings. But sometimes letters, local records, journal articles, biographies, etc. can help build up a picture too, as more than one of the chapters in this volume shows.

A question likely to arise in the minds of many readers is where this volume and the approach exemplified in it stands in relation to the classic history of nursing by Brian Abel-Smith.[5] That work was and is quite distinct from much of what is written as nursing history. First, it is a work by a non-nurse, and it is informed by interests quite other than those pursued in previously published work. Secondly, it is a work which makes extensive use of primary sources, most notably official reports and medical, nursing and administrative journals. Thirdly, it develops a new line of argument and one which in a number of crucial respects is critical of the goals and aspirations of nurses, both singly and as an organised collectivity. Subsequent writers, and those in this volume are no exception, are indebted to Abel-Smith and rely heavily on the work he has done.

Abel-Smith does not fit easily into the category of conventional history as described here. But the interesting thing is that he tends to be treated that way. His book has become, and justifiably so, a set text and an authority in the field. It is easy to see it, not as *a* history, but as *the* history, of nursing. A careful reading of the introductory material shows, however, that for Abel-Smith himself his is a partial history — one governed by a limited set of questions, and producing a limited set of answers. It is a study, he says at the very outset, of the politics of nursing, and it is clear that he means macro-politics more than micro-politics, national-level struggles more than local ones. It is a study too of general nursing — perhaps we should more properly say, above all else, of hospital nursing. Those who have tried to interest themselves in other kinds of nursing will know just how much the sources are biased towards hospital nursing, how they reflect higher social evaluations of this form of nursing and how hard it is to try to redress this, though Abel-Smith himself does not make this point. There are other limitations too, and again Abel-Smith makes them clear:

> The story is told against the wider background of the changing pattern of medical care, but no attempt is made to provide a history of nursing techniques or of nursing as an activity or skill. Little is said about what it was like at different times to nurse, or be trained as a nurse, or to receive nursing care. What the nurse was taught, who taught her, who examined her are all questions which are left unanswered.[6]

It is a sad fact that the twenty years since Abel-Smith wrote his book have seen little further work on nursing. The questions he lists as unanswered have largely remained so. Although there are encouraging signs that this is now changing, the idea of 'nursing research' is still all too likely to conjure up a picture of the questionnaire and the survey, the researcher in the field rather than the researcher in the library and archive room.

The chapters which follow do not constitute a complete rewriting of nursing history. Some deal with old topics in a new way, others with topics which have hardly begun to be explored at all by any writer. The reader will appreciate that many contributors have relied on Abel-Smith, though none have taken the whole of his account as definitive. A high proportion of the essays are authored or co-authored by people who have themselves practised as nurses and who come to the study of history motivated by a desire to understand the past as a guide to present and future action. Each essay is an original piece of work and, as well as offering a new argument and a new interpretation, each author has attempted to give the reader a glimpse of some of the processes of doing historical research.

It is worth dwelling upon the last point, for it was a deliberate decision on my part to encourage contributors to reflect upon their own research strategies and to discuss the assumptions they were rejecting and the ones they were accepting. I was fortunate in being able to find authors who were prepared to do this; many of them are at an advanced, but not a final, stage of their work. They are thus able to articulate the framework they are using and to exemplify it in action while, at the same time, remaining open to possible further developments and modifications. They strive to remind the reader throughout of the status of their argument and the stage they have reached in theory building. To do this is especially unusual in historical work, but to my mind it is valuable and should be done more often. Whether we call the end result history, social history, sociological history, sociology or whatever, is immaterial, provided that it stimulates and provokes.

The collection opens with a chapter by Christopher Maggs. Readers familiar with Abel-Smith's arguments will be able to relate to this immediately, for it complements the sources he used with other materials and starts to suggest not only that the situation in the provincial hospitals was different in key respects from that in the metropolis, but that metropolitan actions were perhaps also in some way influenced by this. His highly justifiable preoccupation with evidence is echoed in the next chapter, though in a different way. Katherine Williams is concerned to show how popular nursing histories, compiled by doctors and by nurses, diverged in important respects. She tries to get behind these accounts to consider the daily operation of nursing practice in the hospital. Mitchell Dean and Gail Bolton, authors of the next contribution, take a rather different approach. They try to place the development of nursing in the context of much more general ideas available in the period — ideas about poverty, about classes, etc. Such ideas are much less far removed from nursing than we would at first expect.

These first three chapters all deal in their different ways with the same well-recognised problem, namely the character of nursing reform in general hospitals in the nineteenth century. Other chapters pursue different themes. My own chapter deals with nurse education, comparing and contrasting the position as it has developed in two different societies, using each to illuminate the other. Such cross-cultural comparison is rare in this field, but does have a distinct contribution to make. The following two chapters have in common an interest in trade unionism among nurses. Mick Carpenter is concerned with psychiatric nursing. He not only underlines the point that it has been neglected but starts to suggest why this was so. He goes on to uncover material about terms and conditions of work and to show how a trade union perspective could emerge and could be sustained in the period before 1914. Paul Bellaby and Patrick Oribabor, by contrast, are concerned with more recent history. Pressures to professionalise and to unionise are their subject-matter and they go back to the 1930s in their search for an understanding of today's trends.

Margaret Connor Versluysen has a different point of entry altogether. She deals with the work of women in healing and deliberately ranges over a much wider timespan and over a much broader scope of healing activities than do other contributors. This chapter should not be seen as standing entirely on its own. The themes she addresses are present, albeit in a more oblique and muted form, at least in the chapters by Maggs, Williams and Carpenter. The last contribution deals directly with the question of available sources and access to them. Janet Foster and Julia Sheppard are both trained archivists and have collaborated on this piece of work in a deliberate effort to open the eyes of would-be researchers to the range of sources they might use.

From the earliest stage of planning this collection of essays, I had aimed to close the volume with a comment and a reaction from someone who was not a doer but a user of nursing history, someone concerned, in the main, more with the future than with the past in nursing. Charlotte Kratz took up this challenge and in the Epilogue she discusses, *inter alia*, the uses, as she sees them, of research of this sort.

A word is perhaps necessary at this point on my decision, as editor, to interject a brief comment at the head of each chapter. I have not used the space in exactly the same way each time. Usually I have taken the opportunity to give some advance warning of what is to come and to emphasise what I see to be the most interesting themes. Sometimes I have suggested lines of criticism, and sometimes I have pointed to linkages between the chapters. I have been deliberately brief and even, at times, deliberately provocative. I have left things unsaid and half-said. My aim has been to open up a debate, to bring others into the process of rewriting nursing history, rather than to foreclose debate by detailed commentary.

This book has been compiled in the conviction that there is much more work to be done in the history of nursing. The results will never be a definitive account but different accounts, prompted by different questions at different times. The challenge of rewriting our history is a continuing task and the better we understand this, the more useful our historical work will be.

Notes

1. Gamp still appears in modern dictionaries as a colloquial term for an umbrella. Mrs Gamp in *Martin Chuzzlewit* is a character much referred to by nursing historians and contributors to this volume are no exception.

2. B. Bailyn, *Education in the Forming of American Society* (University of North Carolina Press, Chapel Hill, 1960), p. 8.

3. H. Butterfield, *The Whig Interpretation of History* (1931) (G. Bell and Sons, London, 1963), p. v.

4. E. P. Thompson, *The Making of the English Working Class* (Penguin Books, Harmondsworth, 1968). See also G. W. Stocking Jr, 'The Limits of "Presentism" and "Historicism" in the Historiography of the Behavioural Sciences' (editorial), *Journal of the History of Behavioural Sciences*, 1 (1965).

5. B. Abel-Smith, *A History of the Nursing Profession* (Heinemann, London, 1960).

6. Ibid., p. xi.

2 NURSE RECRUITMENT TO FOUR PROVINCIAL HOSPITALS 1881–1921

Christopher Maggs

In this chapter Christopher Maggs urges a reassessment of the conventional image of the turn-of-the-century nurse. Was she the mature woman with a vocation for nursing? Was nursing 'something special' in the way of the women attracted to it? Maggs has based his inquiries on hospital records. He has found that these are incomplete and are ambiguous; they do not always relate in a straightforward way to the line of questioning pursued by the historian and must be used with sensitivity. This point is taken up later in this volume by Sheppard and Foster in their discussion of archives. He has also had to use his own analytical skills on a large number of occasions, finding new ways of classifying his data, before he can interpret them, and challenging the taken-for-granted periods into which history is divided.

Christopher Maggs is careful not to claim too much for an arbitrary sample of four hospitals and is right to be cautious. At the same time, his data should give pause for thought, especially when historians have already cautioned that local employment patterns are too diverse to make generalisations for a group or for a time justifiable. Whether or not one accepts Maggs's conclusions about the nurse recruit, his insistence that we should not confuse the ideals of a period with the realities of practice is a point well taken. Furthermore, it becomes especially clear in this chapter that history does not speak for itself.

—————Ed.

Introduction

Scholarship in nursing history has tended to fall into two categories: either a wide-ranging 'history' of the development of nursing as it appears today, or else an attempt to link the development of nursing to related sociological themes, particularly to the notion of professionalism and most recently to patriarchy as an explanation for nursing ideology.[1] This chapter argues that, while overviews are of significant value in the study of nursing history, they fail to take account of the complexities and convolutions which mark out this occupation for women. Such overviews, like those which deal with women's history and women's work,[2] ignore, for the sake of generalisations and 'models', the specific population and labour characteristics which existed, and they do so at the expense of a full appreciation of the 'peculiarities of the English'.[3]

Just as the employment and population patterns in England were essentially local and regional in nature throughout the nineteenth and early twentieth centuries, so we need to consider nursing in the same light, especially if the occupation is to be set in its historical and occupational context. An absence of local information, which would allow such a study to take place and which in turn would enhance the wider historical analysis of nursing, has prompted this preliminary exercise, designed not only to provide some of the missing data, but also to suggest one method of research into nursing in the period.

The data on which this study is based come from a reading of the nurses' registers and matrons' report books in four provincial hospitals: Manchester, Leeds, Southampton and Portsmouth. Three of these were poor law infirmaries, the fourth (Manchester) a voluntary hospital. These hospitals were chosen not only because they kept such records, but also because they provide a provincial balance to the metropolitan experiences more usually described. The work opportunities available to women in these areas not only differed from those in London, but differed again in each locality. Manchester and Leeds offered employment for women in the staple trades of women's work (e.g. textiles), while in Portsmouth and Southampton the predominant opportunities were domestic service, some workshop employment and commercial work such as shop assistants and petty clerical workers.

Although the sources used here provide information about other sections of the hospital nursing staff, this study will concentrate on the evidence about the probationer nurses. While a numerically small section of the total nursing population, locally and nationally, this group is important because a study of origins, education and social backgrounds can lead us to understand not only the 'appeal' of the occupation in general, but also, for example, the way in which nurse probationers' education altered in response to the type of recruit who entered the occupation, and the way in which nursing practice needed to take account of the characters of the nurses involved. Of particular concern in this chapter will be an analysis of the way in which the image of the nurse was produced and used to enhance the status of those who remain in the occupation. Should further local studies confirm the picture built up here, it will mean a serious challenge to the models of the nurse which pervaded the contemporary nursing world, and which seem to persist today. This chapter attempts to pose this challenge by showing the interdependence of two accounts of the probationer nurse in the period, i.e. the 'descriptive' and the 'prescriptive'. While they are treated separately in the text for convenience, it is their 'dialectical' relationship which underlies this analysis.

The Prescriptive Account of the Probationer Nurse

In the late nineteenth century, accounts of nurses in the popular press, in anthologies about women and women's work and in the nursing and medical journals presented an idealised picture when compared with the experiences of contemporaries in the work situation.[4] These accounts were pervasive and fulfilled an important function, not only for the nursing world but for a much wider audience, in particular the patient. These stylised and idealised images may be held to have been prescriptive rather than descriptive: that is, they represented attempts, deliberate and non-deliberate, to erect a model of behaviour, expectations and performance to which all nurses could aspire and subscribe, but they also formed the basis of the criteria by which nurses and nursing might be judged. In particular, they could be used as a yardstick against which new recruits might be measured. While their roots lay in contemporary nurse experience (recruitment, training, practice), these images did not, in important aspects, constitute accurate descriptions of the nurse recruits of the day, as the local evidence will show.

It was felt by contemporary nurses that the optimum age range for applying for nurse training was between 25 and 35 years of age. The sources seem unanimous in arguing that full physical development and growth for a woman was attained only after the twenty-first year. This age group, 25–35, was the one preferred because:

> the necessary responsibilities of the world make it most desirable that those who undertake it [nursing] should be sufficiently mature to face the problems of life and death, disease and sorrow to be found in every ward, even amongst young children.[5]

By the age of 35 years, the woman's ability to adapt to new situations and to ingest new impressions was felt to be waning quickly; at the same time, the older a woman was, the less likely was she able to endure the hard work and long hours, especially of night duty, which made up the contemporary nurse's life.

The probationer was also assumed to be a 'christian lady', displaying those womanly qualities which Sidney Holland once described as making nurses 'the handmaidens of the medical men'.[6] The probationer was expected to undertake a training which would involve her in hard and often unpleasant physical labour, to which she would not have been accustomed. However, as one probationer wrote in

1893, the training,

> in the sense that nurses require it, embraces habits of order
> cleanliness, gentleness and quietness: without these, the theoretical
> training would be worth nothing, *and no true woman* would object
> to scouring, provided it was for the good of the patient . . . *no*
> *woman of refinement of any feeling* would deem it degrading . . .
> (my emphasis)[7]

The home background of the recruit was important in the making of
a nurse and, while some girls were urged to take up charity work as a
prelude to nursing, most were advised by the contemporary literature
to stay at home under their mothers' wings and there continue their
education, at the same time learning the more 'practical' arts of cookery,
needlework and household management. While it was acknowledged
that the gap between leaving school and starting as a nurse was long,
few contemporaries gave positive advice on how to spend that time, in
other than the most general terms. Fewer still seemed to acknowledge
that the recruit might have already been at work in some other
occupation.[8] As for formal education, the sources once again appear
vague, rarely defining what constituted a good educational standard at
which the would-be nurse should aim. In 1898, Chelsea Poor Law
Infirmary required a 'fair education', while Manchester Royal
Infirmary expected recruits to be 'well educated'. Many hospitals and
infirmaries gave would-be nurses an entrance test on general knowledge,
unless they could offer 'acceptable evidence of equivalent examination'.[9] As we shall see, this ambiguity and haziness goes part of the way
towards explaining some of the comments found in the hospital records
about women who left nursing.

This is a brief and selective introduction to the prescriptive model of
the probationer; nevertheless, it does reveal what was part of the
working ideology for contemporary nursing at all levels of the
hierarchy. Such imagery undoubtedly impinged on the ideas held by
other groups (doctors, patients) concerning nurses and nursing. It was
certainly in the mind of the matron as she set about interviewing the
prospective trainee[10] and it influenced the girl who was contemplating
nursing as a career, as both oral evidence and other contemporary
sources show.[11] This prescriptive account therefore forms a useful
framework against which to pose the data from a local study of nurse
recruitment.

The Local Study of Nurse Recruits

A relatively small local study does not enable us to erect alternative historical explanations for the development of nursing; what it can do, however, is to indicate trends and tendencies (e.g. in patterns of recruitment). More specifically, it can raise questions of which future accounts of the development of nursing will need to be aware. When we have presented the evidence from the local study, we will be better able to identify some of these trends and tendencies. Before we can look at this study, however, we need to consider briefly one of the questions which this approach to the study of nursing history raises – the problem of periodisation.

Periodisation is not merely a convenience for the arrangement of material for analysis, for the use of specific time periods assumes there is an intrinsic logic in so doing. In nursing, the logic has commonly been derived from a 'politics of nursing' approach, most obvious in Abel-Smith's attention to the power relationships between elite groups in the process of professionalisation. Such a periodisation seems to take the form 'pre-Nightingale', 'post-Nightingale', 'post-Registration'. While this may answer the questions posed by such an approach to history, neither the approach nor the periodisation is of use if we are interested in the rank-and-file nurse, rather than a small elite group. If we ask who the 'ordinary' nurse was, how she was trained and so on, we need to look for an alternative periodisation, one in which the people involved are seen as agents in social change and as participants in the developments within their work.[12]

Identifying important and significant periods which take this alternative concern into account is a difficult and evolving task: difficult because, until more detailed research has been carried out which looks at these issues and these 'ordinary' people, definite eras cannot be established. As a preliminary exercise, in the spirit of what can only be a preliminary paper, designed to question the current periodisation rather than produce an alternative, we would suggest that the following division, 1881–1914 and 1914–1921, will serve its purpose.

At the end of the nineteenth century, the growth in the institutional care of the sick, both in voluntary and in public hospitals and infirmaries, brought with it an increased demand for nurses. This 'take-off' may be illustrated in Table 2.1, which shows that the increase in hospitals (expressed here in terms of hospital beds) dates from the latter part of the century rather than the earlier (or even 'Nightingale') period, 1850–1875.

Table 2.1: Average Annual Increase in Hospital Beds, 1861–1921
(England and Wales)

	1861–91	1891–1911	1911–12
Voluntary hospitals	492	685	1,333
Public hospitals	1,108	3,552	1,773
Totals	1,600	4,237	3,106

Source: taken and modified from R. Pinker, *English Hospital Statistics, 1861–1938* (Heinemann, London, 1966), Table 1, p. 51.

Besides the absolute increase in the numbers of nurses required by this institutional expansion, the period from 1881 up to the outbreak of the First World War marks a qualitative change in attitudes towards sickness and towards those who cared for the sick. The growth of a 'nursing' literature, journals and even novels served to reflect this change, and the issues raised by this new awareness (which was capitalised upon with some effect by sections of the nursing elite[13]) became public property and concern.[14]

In this period, 1881–1913, the most significant quantitative change in nursing was the rapid expansion of the poor law sector, in which (following from the Poor Law Order of 1897) both the numbers of infirmaries and the numbers of nurses increased considerably. The need to provide establishments of trained nurses in these infirmaries, and hence the need to recruit and train their own probationers, saw the development of separate training programmes in the public sector and the stirrings of a rivalry between the poor law training hospitals and the voluntary hospitals which still exists today, long after the distinctions have passed.

Attempts to keep what labour there was available in nursing, at a time of a general shortage of women in many service sector employments, constituted one factor in the introduction of the three-year training scheme in both sectors during this period, 1881–1914, and a written contract of employment for probationers was almost universal by the turn of the century.

Turning to the period from 1914 to 1921, no account of nursing or of any other occupation can fail to take into consideration the effects of the First World War and the immediate post-war period. Not only did the war bring about the additional burden to the health services of war casualties; it also highlighted the fact that nursing was geared to the care of a civilian population, whose rapid recovery was not a necessary corollary of treatment. The rapid turn-round of military patients was essential in the pre-conscription years, to replace the enormous losses at the front. Lack of numbers to care for this increased patient-load, at home and in the Services and their auxiliary units, allowed the charitable organisations, such as the Red Cross, to involve themselves at the highest level in nursing planning, while at the level of the individual institution Red Cross volunteers began helping out in the wards quite early on in the war. More vexatious to the nursing elite (and some rank-and-file nurses), the appearance of Voluntary Aid Detachment (VAD) nurses challenged the established nurse-training patterns, the type of women recruited as nurses, the discipline and the *modus vivendi* which the nursing establishment had so painstakingly sought to build up. The shortage of nurses, to which we have already alluded, was further complicated by the wider range of alternative employments open to women, as we shall see from the local data. While the period ends effectively with the passing of the Nurses' Registration Act, 1919, and its implementation, the period 1914–1921 is more usefully considered here for its relationship to the changes which war made in women's work and in nursing itself. Such a periodisation as this can, therefore, not only take account of the quantitative changes in nursing throughout the entire period, but also set these in relationship to the qualitative changes which occurred, permitting an understanding of nursing as it was practised by the women involved.

Using this periodisation, we can ask specific questions of our local sources, in order to build up a picture of the sort of women who became nurses in each time period. For the sake of brevity and clarity, I have chosen five areas of analysis: namely, number of recruits, ages, previous work experience, mobility and leaving patterns. Clearly questions such as the educational standard of the recruit, religious affiliation, and aspirations or motives for nursing would need to be examined for a complete study.

Number of Recruits

Nationally (England and Wales) the numbers of women employed in nursing in any capacity were 35,216 in 1881, 53,003 in 1891, 64,209 in 1901, 77,055 in 1911 and 110,039 in 1921. These numbers are not absolutely comparable, in view of the classification changes which took place at many censuses, particularly the 1921 census. However, the over-all trend of a significant increase in absolute numbers is indisputable.[15]

This national trend was repeated at the local level and in the individual hospitals. Manchester Royal Infirmary took on 1,566 new probationers between 1881 and 1921; Portsmouth Poor Law Infirmary took on 439 in the shorter period that it existed as a training hospital (1905–1921). The Leeds Poor Law Infirmary and the Southampton Poor Law Infirmary, which began training probationers in 1895 and 1902 respectively, engaged 514 and 332 new recruits up to 1921.

The total numbers of new recruits to an individual hospital varied with the size of the hospital and its nursing establishment. The hospital records, however, do suggest that the largest increase of probationers came in the war period, when each was wholly or in part taken over as a military hospital. Before that time, only marginal increases in the yearly intake of probationers are detectable in the data, despite increases either in the over-all size of the hospitals or in the bed-usage rates. The same records also suggest that there were relatively few 'trained' nurses per probationer throughout the entire period of this study, as was the case in the occupation as a whole.[16]

Taken together, these two features of probationer numbers and ratios of trained to untrained nurses point to a cost-conscious service where the labour force was largely unqualified and inexperienced. Even when the total numbers of probationers (and volunteers) rose during the war period, the ratios of nurses to patients and nurses to untrained recruits remained fairly constant.

Ages of Recruits to Nursing

There existed no formal, i.e. legal, constraints on the age of entry for new recruits to nursing throughout the period. Such age limits as did exist were more the result of contemporary attitudes, quasi-scientific beliefs and the exigencies of the service. As a general rule, women were said by contemporaries to be recruited for training in hospitals and infirmaries in the 25–35 age range (see above), but if we look at the local evidence a different picture emerges.

In Leeds Poor Law Infirmary, in every year, a majority of recruits were aged over 21 and under 25 (80 per cent of all recruits) and only after 1920 were any significant numbers of under-21s recruited. The exception was in 1915, the first year after the war began, when they first appeared and formed 10 per cent of all recruits in that year. While some of these under-21s were so close to their twenty-first birthdays that they could be classed in the next age bracket (21–25), others were undoubtedly well under the age of 21, although never younger than 19 years of age. In all the years for which records exist, no probationer was over 35, and few (less than 20 per cent in all years) were over 31 years of age. Whether or not the result of policy, the general age range of applicants, or specific local employment patterns, the general pattern established at the Leeds Poor Law Infirmary was to recruit principally from within the 21–25 age group throughout our period.

This pattern was repeated at the Manchester Royal Infirmary, although here the proportion of 21–25-year-olds was less, approximately 60 per cent over-all, falling in individual years to less than 50 per cent of all recruits. A greater proportion of 26–30-year-olds was recruited to Manchester Royal Infirmary, 30 per cent over-all, while a number of older entrants, i.e. over 31 years of age, was consistently recruited. In a fifth of all years, more over-25s were engaged than under-25s, although the majority of all recruits were still under 30. As at Leeds Poor Law Infirmary, the under-21s were not engaged, for whatever reasons, until the end of the First World War, and then only in small numbers. Significantly, the slightly lower proportion of girls aged 21–25 was found only at Manchester Royal Infirmary, the one voluntary hospital considered in this paper. It might be that the higher age of entry described in the prescriptive model had some firm basis in the policies of the voluntary hospitals, although the specific local employment patterns for women's work in general need to be considered before making a final judgement.

At first sight, Portsmouth Poor Law Infirmary appears to have had its own recruiting pattern, in which a proportion of all entrants in each year was under 21 years of age. Before 1914, this proportion ranged from 3 to 20 per cent, but at the onset of war it began to rise, from 30 per cent in 1914 to 60 per cent in 1920. Also, before 1914 most recruits had been over 21 and under 30, and none was over 35, although an average of 4 per cent each year were aged between 31 and 35. Over all, however, if we include the under-21s, Portsmouth Poor Law Infirmary pursued a policy very much like the general trend we have already noted, i.e. that of recruiting a majority of probationers aged 25 years and under.

In confirmation of the increased availability of the younger (i.e. under-21) female worker at the end of the war and in the early post-war period, the number of applicants for posts as probationer at Portsmouth Poor Law Infirmary in this age group rose, from approximately 10 per cent throughout the war to 25 per cent in 1918, 50 per cent in 1919 and 54 per cent in 1920. Most of these were actually engaged as probationers, and this took place as the total number of applicants in the 21–25 age group fell from 60 per cent to 27 per cent of all applicants between 1918 and 1921. The explanation for this shift is complex, involving considerations of a released workforce (i.e. released from war work), attitude changes, displacement in other occupations, altered marriage patterns and local employment opportunities, all of which will require further investigation in order fully to understand the effects of war on women's work and on nursing in the twentieth century.

We can begin to see, however, even from these limited data, that the actual recruit was a younger woman than the one portrayed in the nursing literature, aged between 21 and 25 years, and that it was the war period, when competition for labour became acute, which accelerated the change to the acceptance as recruits of women aged under 21 years.

Previous Work Experiences of Recruits to Nursing

The presentation of this section of the local evidence is made difficult as there is a lack of data for Southampton Poor Law Infirmary and gaps in the data available from the other hospitals, and because of the general problems of collating the diverse employment opportunities available to women in the period. The data do provide an opportunity, however, to attempt an alternative descriptive classification of the work in which probationers had previously been engaged. This classification is not linked to industries or trades; instead it takes note of the similarities and relationships between and across work carried out by women. Thus, for example, it is suggested that shopwork and waitressing can be grouped together because in each there is a common and significant element of client–worker relationship (involving deference, manners, dress and so on) which is absent, for example, from factory work, where timekeeping and speed of working are more important, both to employer and employee, than personal appearances. The list in Table 2.2 is therefore an attempt to give a general descriptive classification of those occupations in which nurse recruits had engaged prior to nursing, a classification which sets nursing firmly within the context of other areas of women's work. Using this classification, the available data from our local sources are presented in Figure 2.1, where for each period the percentage of recruits following a particular category of work described above is shown.

Using this classification, Figure 2.1 shows that throughout the entire period, 1881–1921, the highest proportion of all recruits came from Categories 1 and 2, i.e. from among women who had no previous occupation, or from among women who had already worked in some capacity as nurses. The number of recruits who had previous work

Table 2.2: Classification of Previous Occupations of Recruits

1. Nil	This corresponds to those whom the Census gives as 'Unoccupied', especially those women in the younger age groups. In the local hospital evidence, this category includes such entries as 'None', 'At Home', 'Nil'.
2. Nursing	This category includes fever nurses, asylum nurses, monthly and village nurses, mental nurses, cottage-hospital nurses in children's hospitals, attendants and in some cases (particularly after 1902) midwives. In other words, this group represents the number of women who had worked and had called themselves 'nurse', in some capacity, and who were now wanting to train or retrain as 'general nurse'.
3. Domestic service and 4. Personal services	These are two distinct groups, but are better seen in relationship to each other than treated in separate sections. There are important drawbacks to using the census categories of domestic service; for example, it was well known that a companion or lady's maid would provide a different type of service from a parlourmaid or housemaid (despite abuses of the distinctions) and be involved in a different sort of relationship with the employer, one based not on a hierarchical arrangement of function and duties, but rather on a working distinction between the provision of an 'hotel' service and the provision of a 'privatised' service. Hence, in the former group are such occupations as cook, housekeeper, maid, etc. and in the latter are wet-nursing, children's nurses, nannies, governesses, nursemaids and companions.
5. Clerical and Public service work	Included under this heading are those occupations such as bookkeeper, cashier, stenographer, telephonist, post office worker, and assistant (i.e. unqualified) librarian.
6. Clothing and textile work	This category takes account of those traditional areas of women's employment in workshops and factories, for example milling machinist, dressmaker, weaver, seamstress.
7. Shopwork	Shopwork includes here waitresses, shop assistants and women whose work was noted by contemporaries for its face-to-face dealings with clients, which involved the worker in considerations of dress, manners and so on.
8. Education	This category covers pupil teachers, elementary teachers and private teachers (except governesses) who had some degree of training. Also this category would include women who taught music or other 'arts' on a private basis.
9. War work and miscellaneous employment	This residual group includes those jobs which were directly created or made open to women by the war, in e.g. land army, VAD work (non-nursing), munitions, tram conducting, and also the very small number of trades such as artist and photographer which appear in the post-war period.

Figure 2.1: Percentage of Probationers from each Employment Category, in Three Provincial Hospitals (various dates)[a]

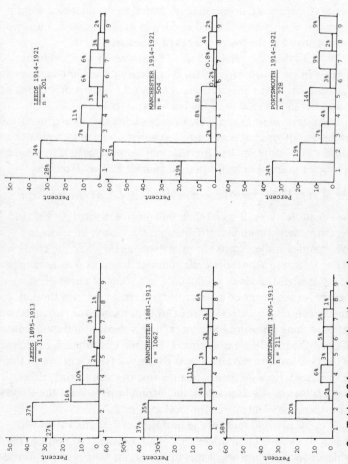

a. See Table 2.2 for an explanation of each group.

experience exceeded those who had none (except at Portsmouth Poor Law Infirmary in its early years of probationer training). For the entire period, the most significant recruitment area was Category 2 (i.e. 'nurses'), in particular this was the case at Manchester Royal Infirmary, where the prestige of training in a voluntary hospital, or the local competition for private cases from Manchester Royal Infirmary-trained nurses, may have encouraged a higher proportion of women to retrain there.

As the figure shows, the recruitment of ex-domestic servants by these hospitals was never significant (except to Leeds Poor Law Infirmary in the early years of probationer training), and the trend was towards an over-all decline in the number of recruits from domestic service (Category 3), in part due, no doubt, to the increased recruitment of women who had been working in shops, engaged in war work and employed in the lower reaches of education.

While all three hospitals recruited from women who had been engaged in war work, after 1918, Portsmouth's peculiarity as a garrison town and naval base probably accounts for the highest proportion of recruits from this section of the female workforce.

In general, while in each year or each period there was a significant proportion of girls entering nursing as a first occupation, a greater number of recruits had had previous employment, even if this had been in another hospital or institution, or another branch of nursing.

The Mobility of Female Labour as it Affected Nurse Recruitment

Two major features of social change in nineteenth-century England were urbanisation and industrialisation: the growth of urban communities at the expense of rural depopulation, and the creation of a labour force and set of social relationships determined and disciplined by the capitalist mode of production. In a study of nursing history these processes might be expected to give rise to the migration of female workers to centres of urban growth, themselves associated with the provision of health care services (both voluntary and state financed), and perhaps to an increasing emphasis on the institutional, as opposed to the personal and privatised, care of the sick (see Dean and Bolton in this volume). Here we focus upon the first of these factors, although they are inseparable in practice, the second being beyond the scope of the evidence available from our local sources.

In order to avoid some of the problems of definition as to what constitutes a rural or an urban area[17] and somewhat to simplify the evidence for the purposes of this summary, the origins of the recruits will be organised as follows.

Local Recruits.   These recruits came from the city or town in which they now worked as nurses in training, i.e. Leeds, Southampton, Portsmouth and Manchester. Also included are those women who travelled less than 25 miles to come and train in these hospitals: that is, women who came from the area dominated to some significant degree by the nearby town or city, the urban 'sphere of influence'.

Rural Recruits.   Such recruits were living in small communities and villages outside of the areas of influence noted above. While the geography of England puts few such communities outside of any urban sphere, the important feature here is that the women went to a hospital in a distant urban area to train, and not the one closest to their home.

Urban Recruits.   These recruits came from other urban centres, towns and cities.

Immigrant Recruits.   Such recruits came from Ireland, Wales, Scotland and, in a few cases, from outside Great Britain, e.g. Canada.

The available local evidence is summarised in Table 2.3. We should note that each of the urban areas covered, i.e. Leeds, Southampton and Portsmouth, enjoyed an expanding population, particularly of females, during the pre-war period, after which the picture is somewhat distorted because of wartime conditions.

The patterns as between the hospitals are strikingly different, more so perhaps in the earlier period than the later one. With one exception, however, we should note that they do recruit heavily from outside their own local area.

In terms of trends over time, the only similarity between hospitals apparent from this table is the increase in the number of recruits from outside England. The majority of these came from Ireland (from 11 to 30 per cent at Leeds Poor Law Infirmary; 6–21 per cent at Portsmouth Poor Law Infirmary; and 18–21 per cent at Southampton Poor Law Infirmary). At the Leeds Infirmary these women were recruited as recruitment from all other areas fell; at the Southampton Infirmary, few women were recruited from other urban areas and this seems to have been offset by the engagement of Irish women; while the losses to local war work in Portsmouth might well explain the recruitment of Irish girls there. Southampton Infirmary increased its recruitment a

Table 2.3: Origins of Recruits to Three Provincial Hospitals, 1881–1921, as a Percentage of all Recruits

Recruits	before 1913[a]					1914–1921				
	Local	Rural	Urban	Immi-grant	No.	Local	Rural	Urban	Immi-grant	No.
Hospital:										
Leeds	38%	42%	9%	11%	313	28%	37%	5%	30%	201
Southampton	39%	16%	27%	18%	164	49%	18%	12%	21%	168
Portsmouth	68%	18%	8%	6%	211	47%	19%	13%	21%	228

a. For information on precise dates covered see Figure 2.1.

little from within its own 'sphere of influence' (39–49 per cent), unlike the other two hospitals, and this reflected the general expansion which the town of Southampton underwent in the period. At the same time, the proportion of immigrant recruits, i.e. Irish, Welsh and Scots, started at 18 per cent as the highest of the four, but increased only a little.

The over-all picture which emerges is that which one would expect from other studies of migration and which corresponds to models of short-distance migration, especially of women.[18] The figures for the war period are difficult to interpret, but their significance probably lies in the numbers of recruits who came from Ireland, Wales and to a lesser extent from Scotland, and who began to appear in all areas during and immediately after this time. Such an influx does not appear to have been commented upon in either the contemporary or subsequent accounts of nursing, but their obvious presence and recruitment must contribute to any future discussion about the supply of nurses in the period.

Reasons Given for Leaving Training Hospital, Before and After Completion of Training

The only hospital for which evidence is available for this topic is Southampton Poor Law Infirmary. Most of the statements in the surviving records are subjective, frequently vague, and often ambiguous.[19] Table 2.4 attempts to quantify what evidence there is from this source as to why women gave up nursing.

The numbers of nurses who left because they had qualified fell by 11 per cent and never exceeded much more than half of all nurses who left in the period 1905–21. More nurses left because of an expressed dislike of the work or because they were said by the matron to be unsuitable for training. While there was very little increase in the

Table 2.4: Reasons Given for Leaving Nursing, During or After
Training (Southampton Poor Law Infirmary)

Reason given	1905–13	1914–21
	%	%
Completion of training	54	43
Dislike of nursing	16	29
Ill health	12	11
'Ran away'; 'failed to return to duty'; 'left without permission'	6	6
Failed examinations	4	4
Marriage	1	5
Family reasons: either ill health or required at home	3	2
Dismissed	3	2
To take up other nursing work	1	3
Total number	211	228

numbers of women who wanted to train in a voluntary hospital rather
than a poor law infirmary, there was a slightly larger increase in the
numbers who left to be married, this increase occurring in the later war
years, when the hospital was used by the military authorities. The
relatively high proportion of women who left for health reasons must
be viewed in the light of the type of patients treated and the nursing
and medical skills then available. However, in some instances the health
problem was related more to the physical and mental stress brought
about by the work itself, for example flat feet, varicose veins and
nervous debility, this at a time when the medical test before starting
training had become universal practice and more strict in its application.

The length of stay in the job is naturally related to the reasons given
for leaving, but again the data are incomplete on this interesting point.
From the Southampton and Portsmouth Infirmaries, however (and
particularly from the Southampton Infirmary records), a picture
emerges of a constant stream throughout the entire year of women
beginning and leaving training. Some seem to have stayed for only one
day, a week or a month, and while some of this exodus may be
attributed to a desire to weed out the 'unfit' and the 'undesirable', it
still appears a formidable indictment of the method of recruitment. An
average stay in post seems to have been between one and a half and
two years, which suggests that only half, if that many, of all recruits to
Southampton Poor Law Infirmary actually completed their training
there. Whether they went on to take their training elsewhere, to
practise as 'unqualified' nurses or were effectively lost to the occupation is unclear at this stage, and will only be clarified when further

local studies have been carried out.

To sum up, local evidence about specific recruit characteristics suggests that the actual recruit differed in important respects from the 'prescriptive' model as it appeared in contemporary literature. The probationer was undoubtedly a younger person than the model allowed, and she was becoming younger as the occupation developed, bringing it into direct competition for labour power with other areas of women's work. Far from being a first or even prime career choice, this ideologically dominant sector of nursing drew upon women already experienced in work and wage discipline,[20] and if hospital nursing and probationer training offered a degree of occupational mobility to some women, it also played some part in the geographical mobility of female labour in the period. Although there are important gaps in our knowledge about the origins of recruits and their motives for moving, this study has suggested that hospital training could be one small 'pull-factor' in encouraging women to leave home and seek work in the urban areas.[21] Further studies will be necessary before this mobility is fully understood; in particular such studies will need to ask whether it was nursing itself, or the specific institution, or the attraction of a particular town or city, which provided the prime element in the geographical mobility of nurse recruits.

It is clear, then, that there is a need for local and regional factors to be included in an account of the development of nursing. Studies which perceive nursing to be a unitary occupation, even in a restricted sense (e.g. the poor law nursing service), ignore important features in the history of nursing and the study of occupations and work. This preliminary study offers some suggestions as to how such local studies might be undertaken, using the records of the hospitals themselves.

It was argued at the beginning of the chapter, however, that it is not the contrasts and contradictions which emerge when the two accounts are put together which, important as they are, form the major contribution which studies like this one can make. Rather, it is the interdependence of the two models, the prescriptive and the descriptive, which offers the most interest to the historian. How was it that an 'ideal-type' nurse might emerge when the actual recruit seldom attained even a passing similarity to the ideal? Why was nursing concerned with status imagery and professional organisation, and what effects did the actual type of recruit have on these concerns? In the last part of this study we turn to this discussion and, using specific recruit characteristics already discussed, examine how the two models could exist side by side, without apparent confusion.

Discussion

The key to the prescriptive model of the nurse was the commitment by the woman to nursing, to the exclusion of all other considerations. The model therefore concerned itself primarily with what sort of women became nurses, and in particular it sought to emphasise nursing as a career chosen after mature reflection by women for whom material considerations (including marriage) were of minimal importance or, even better still, were rejected in favour of nursing. The age at which such decisions were made, and the procedure by which the right sort of woman was selected and the wrong sort rejected, were important aspects of this dialectical process; the local material presented here enables us to discuss these areas in more detail.

Linking many aspects of the idealised model of the nurse entrant, as presented in the first part of this chapter, were quasi-scientific beliefs which, although superseded as science developed, were tenaciously subscribed to in the contemporary nursing world. We have seen, for example, that the prescribed age of entry was 25–35 years, whereas the local evidence suggests that most recruits came from the 21–25 age range. Phrases in the contemporary sources refer to the candidates' 'maturity', 'full development' and so on, and are presented in a scientific manner. Attempts to discover the basis of these statements in contemporary science prove difficult, unless one is prepared to look at the decades before our time period, and even as far back as the early years of the nineteenth century. Many of these apparently scientific statements about human development were being effectively challenged by natural and biological scientists,[22] and we find that, while there is, inevitably, a time-lag between scientific advancement and changes in popular beliefs about those ideas, not only were these statements about nurses made at the beginning of our period, circa 1881, but they were in evidence in the war and post-war periods as well, and this in an occupation in which the elite claimed scientific method as part of its rationale.

These statements, couched in the quasi-scientific language of the day, came not only from the nurses and doctors, but from social scientists and investigators, and several of these wrote confidently of 'the most efficient age periods' in which a woman should work, including working as a nurse.[23] The problem remains, however, of trying to explain the apparent disjuncture between these statements and the actual experiences of the time.

It is possible to suggest that an older woman posed less of a discipline problem than a younger woman. A woman who was unmarried at 25 or 30 had less likelihood of marriage, and was hence more liable to accept the enclosed world of the hospital as a substitute for family life. This cloistered existence was certainly a feature of life for many nurses, as oral evidence has helped to demonstrate,[24] and the added prospect of some pension rights for long service helped to enhance the life-long commitment to nursing for a section of women. Evidently, it was not in the minds of all recruits, as the high wastage rates show, and perhaps these statements about the 'best' age for entry ought to be seen as part of a justification or rationalisation for the experiences of those who actually remained, i.e. the older, unmarried nurses of sister and charge nurse rank.

Indeed, it might be argued that the prescriptive model applied less to the new recruit and more to the nurse who stayed in the occupation. As we have seen, the 'drop-out' rate could be high as 50 per cent in some hospitals, and many of the contemporary statements about nursing and nursing qualities may be seen as explanations of why women chose this cloistered existence, and how in turn they attempted to recruit like-minded individuals into the occupation.

The principal step in that process was when the matron, with the prescriptive model in mind, interviewed the prospective nurse, although some form of preliminary 'weeding-out' exercise may have taken place. This weeding-out was begun by the matron (or committee where it was still in existence for the hiring of nurses), when reading the letters of application or returned application forms. These were often accompanied by a photograph of the applicant, in particular when she lived so far away from the hospital as to be unable to attend for interview. Bad handwriting and incorrect form filling seem to mark out some of the unsuccessful applications; in some cases the 'tone' of the letter could mean that an interview was not offered to the girl, and very occasionally women in certain jobs would not be invited to carry on with their application.[25] There are, in the case of Portsmouth Poor Law Infirmary, examples of women being declined a post on the basis of the photograph alone, which suggests or reinforces the notion that a 'good nurse' could be recognised on sight by the experienced matron. Few of the Irish or Welsh applicants living in their own countries at the time of applying attended for interview, but few were ever refused at least a trial period in the hospital of their choice. There were possibly links between certain hospitals and infirmaries and convents and parish priests in Ireland from whom the hospitals received applications but, on the whole, most of these recruits were still selected on the basis of the photograph and the testimonial.

It remains difficult, however, to explain the subsequent losses of recruits in training, if this selection procedure went on. Contemporary accounts show the importance to the matrons of the interview itself in the enlistment of recruits;[26] it was the time when the model held by the matron who had (considerable) experience of nurses and nursing could be applied in a face-to-face meeting with a potential nurse. Frequently portrayed in the contemporary accounts as a *tête-à-tête* between the stern aunt-like figure of the matron and an eager novitiate, the interview owed more to personal preference and prejudice than any principles of management then available to the senior nurse. Reading between the lines of the local sources, a different picture is suggested – that of a young woman unprepared to be completely overawed by the occasion, having had experiences of being dealt with by other prospective employers, and of a matron who, having written down the candidate's age, religion, educational standard, etc., confined her remarks to hours of duty, behaviour in the nurses' home and articles of uniform to be brought by the recruit on the first day. In other words, the uncertainty of the selection process seems to have revolved around the supposed and expected ability of a matron to recognise on sight a potentially 'good nurse'. That she could not, as the local evidence has suggested, does not at any time seem to have interfered with the practice.

The knowledge in the mind of the matron of the 'discipline' process within nursing and within the individual hospital which could mould the trainee probably prevented any changes being forced upon the selection method. Indeed, it might have been as much an essential exposition of the matron's power as a way of enlisting new recruits, in terms of the hierarchy of the nursing process. Given, then, the initial 'logic' of this procedure, the 'drop-out' rate could be explained by accusing the women who left of having un-nurse-like qualities – laziness, indolence, bad education, a lack of dedicated application, and so forth – qualities, or rather vices, which prevented the woman as an individual from undertaking the essential rigours of hospital work and demonstrating the necessary self-discipline which nursing demanded of its practitioners. This system of accusing those who left of such vices allowed an individualistic approach to the problem of nurse wastage, rather than an explanation couched in collective terms, which might have threatened the occupation by attacking part of its dominant world-view. At the same time, these individualistic explanations were reworked into the collective explanations which served to justify the actions of those who remained within the occupation, at least within the hospital section of the occupation.

In some hospitals, in particular the voluntary hospitals, there were waiting lists of women who wished to train as nurses. The existence of such a potential workforce must have helped in reinforcing these ideas of nurse- and non-nurse-like qualities. This complacency could be and was challenged, as during the war and post-war periods when recruitment of nurses faced competition from other areas in some hospitals. In others, for example Portsmouth Poor Law Infirmary and Southampton Poor Law Infirmary, there were sometimes no women at all on the waiting list. Matrons were forced to advertise, some for the first time, and many had only mixed success. There were occasions from 1913 onwards when demands were made for a lower age of entry, particularly in the poor law sector which faced the brunt of the competition for female labour, but such a change only occurred after the war when the shortage was most acutely felt.

It has been shown that, despite the presumed vocational attitudes characteristic of the occupation as a whole, many women failed to complete their training, and it is possible that this was a general feature of women's employment throughout the period. Such mobility of labour, together with a willingness by the women to move geographically in search of employment, demonstrates the close links which nursing has with other types of women's work in the period. Altogether, it appears that the nurse recruit was much more like her fellow woman worker than we might have gathered from the nursing histories, and that discovering her involves looking beyond nursing itself and towards the study of women in British society.

Acknowledgement

This chapter arises from research undertaken as a postgraduate student at the University of Bath, during 1977–78, with the help of an SSRC grant. I would like to acknowledge the enormous help given to me by June Hannam and Christopher Frayling.

Notes

1. Examples of wide-ranging histories include B. Abel-Smith, *A History of the Nursing Profession* (Heinemann, London, 1960), M. Baly, *Nursing and Social Change* (Macmillan, London, 1973), M. A. Nutting and L. Dock, *A History of Nursing* (Putnam, New York, 1907), 4 vols. Two authors who focus on

professionalism are M. Carpenter, 'The New Managerialism and Professionalism in Nursing', in M. Stacey *et al.* (eds), *Health Care and the Division of Labour* (Croom Helm, London, 1977), and C. Davies, 'Continuities in the Development of Hospital Nursing in Britain', *Journal of Advanced Nursing*, 2 (1977). Patriarchy is discussed in E. Gamarnikow's 'Sexual Division of Labour: the case of Nursing', in A. Kuhn and A. M. Wolpe (eds), *Feminism and Materialism* (Routledge and Kegan Paul, London, 1978).

2. P. Branca, *Women in Europe Since 1750* (Croom Helm, London, 1978); G. Lerner, 'Liberating Women's History', in B. A. Carroll (ed.), *Liberating Women's History: theoretical and critical essays* (University of Illinois Press, Illinois, 1975).

3. This is the title of a well-known essay by E. P. Thompson, first published in the *New Left Review* and recently reprinted in E. P. Thompson (ed.), *The Poverty of Theory* (Merlin Press, London, 1978).

4. For example, Lady S. E. M. Jeune (ed.), *Ladies at Work* (Arnold, London, 1893). See also in the same volume H. and R. Wilson, 'Hospital Nursing'.

5. L. Maule, 'Training Schools and Other Nursing Institutions', in (various authors), *Science and the Art of Nursing* (Cassells, London, n.d.), pp. 48–9. See also M. Voysey, *Nursing: Hints to Probationers* (Scientific Press, London, 1905), and M. Vivian, *Lectures to Nurses in Training* (Scientific Press, London, 1920).

6. Quoted from A. Hughes, 'Nursing as a Vocation', in *Science and the Art of Nursing*, p. 96.

7. W. Brockbank, *History of Nursing at the Manchester Royal Infirmary* (Manchester University Press, Manchester, 1970), p. 65.

8. M. M. Bird, *Women at Work* (Chapman and Hall, London, 1911); Vivian, 'Lectures', *Nursing Times and Midwives Journal* (1905).

9. See H. C. Burdett, *Hospital Gazette* (Scientific Press, London, 1898).

10. Brockbank, *History of Nursing*.

11. Maule, 'Training Schools'.

12. Periodisation is debated fully in Lerner, 'Liberating Women's History'.

13. Mrs Bedford Fenwick's journal, the *Nursing Record*, led the field in editorial comment on the shortage of nurses and the standard of those nurses available to the middle classes in particular.

14. For example, the *Lancet* inquiry into the shortage of nurses which was reported in the daily press, including *The Times*. (See Davies in this volume.)

15. These data are from census returns. Abel-Smith, *Nursing Profession*, gives a full discussion in an appendix to his volume. See also C. Davies, 'Making Sense of the Census in Britain and the USA: the Changing Occupational Classification and the Position of Nurses', *Sociological Review* (forthcoming).

16. Burdett gave figures of 11,038 nurses employed in voluntary hospitals, of whom 1,687 were trained and 7,062 were probationers in 1903. Evidence of Sir H. C. Burdett, *Select Committee on Nurses Registration* (1905), vii, pp. 102–3. See also Abel-Smith, *Nursing Profession*, p. 257, where a ratio of one trained nurse to three students is given.

17. This point is discussed in J. Saville, *Rural Depopulation in England and Wales* (Routledge and Kegan Paul, London, 1957); see especially pp. 59–69.

18. Ibid.

19. For example (Southampton Poor Law Infirmary):

Left after 14 months: 'Disregarded her agreement to serve for 3 years. Very slow in her work and objected to being criticised.'

Left after 3½ years: 'failed to pass her Final Examination: Uneducated and dull in theory. Quick in her practical and good to patients.'

Left after 3 months: 'Flatfooted, much too delicate.'

Left after 1 month: 'Left because her mother was ill.'
Left after 9 months: 'Left to be married. Very uneducated.'
Left after 10 months: 'Quietly impertinent . . . left without permission. Had peroxide hair and appearance not nurse-like . . .'
Dismissed after 3 months: [the only instance of a girl actually being dismissed in these records]: 'Most unsuitable for training as a nurse, conduct unsatisfactory. Appears to have a mania for running up bills which she cannot pay. Found smacking a child and altogether bad tempered. Dismissed.'

20.   See Gamarnikow, 'Sexual Division of Labour'.
21.   See T. McBride, *The Domestic Revolution* (Croom Helm, London, 1976).
22.   The latest in a long line at that time being H. Havelock Ellis, *Man and Woman* (Scott, London, 1904).
23.   Such sentiments seem to have survived in recent social science, e.g. 'the physical and psychological needs of mature men and women were being dealt with in hospitals by young unmarried girls. And at an early age, girls were being faced with the emotional strains of suffering and death.' Abel-Smith, *Nursing Profession*, pp. 124–5.
24.   Several interviewees who had stayed in nursing spoke of having no interests outside of the hospital, and even when they went to concerts and plays, etc., they spoke of these excursions as isolated events taken in the company of other females, especially other nurses: C. Maggs, unpublished oral interviews, 1976–78.
25.   For example, 'Miss A, 21 years old; Wardmaid at Milton Hospital, Portsmouth – Application not entertained'.
26.   Maule, 'Training Schools', p. 52. See also 'Two Letters from a Matron', *Nursing Times*, vol. 1 (1 June 1907).

3 FROM SARAH GAMP TO FLORENCE NIGHTINGALE: A CRITICAL STUDY OF HOSPITAL NURSING SYSTEMS FROM 1840 TO 1897[1]

Katherine Williams

If history does not speak for itself, whose accounts of nursing history should we believe? Katherine Williams shows us that accounts given by nurses and by doctors, while at first sight similar, diverge markedly. Yet each is systematic and each coherent. What she does, most strikingly, is to marshal apparently disparate views into positions essentially intelligible in terms of the interests of the two occupational groups. For herself, she is not prepared to rely uncritically on either account. She searches for what she calls 'alternative evidence', finding it in a variety of source materials and particularly in accounts of the everyday practice of nursing work.

Critics might wish to ponder on her notion of alternative evidence, and ask whether accounts of practice might not be subject to similar biases to accounts of historical development. But if they do this, the author will have succeeded in an important part of her task. Since the lesson, to me at least, is this: do not discard a biased record — its bias is just what is going to help you to understand the tensions of a period.

—————Ed.

We hear a great deal about systems; it seems there was or is an old system, and that there is or will be a new system. Under the former, it is said, all was bad; under the latter, we shall behold perfection.

A Nurse, 'Systems of Nursing',
Edinburgh Medical Journal, May 1880.

Introduction

This chapter is a critical study of a period of nursing which was seen by its historians as one in which the foundations of modern nursing were laid. For these writers, nursing variously progressed during the nineteenth century from a system that was morally bad and inadequate for its purpose to a system that, in the eyes of the nursing historian, required little more by 1897 than that the state should legitimate it. In contrast, the medical historian is disturbed by the remedies that have been introduced and claims that there are many obstacles to such settled public identity.

The task of this chapter is to examine these claims and assess their status as objective history. Written sources relating to nursing will be analysed critically and the evidence they supply will inform the following questions: what are the facts of nineteenth-century hospital nursing and how do they relate to popular nursing histories; do these emerge as fact, or as interpretation of fact?

The historian, E. H. Carr, in his book *What is History?*, deals extensively with these issues of historiography. He argues that, though 'facts and documents are essential to the historian, they do not by themselves constitute history . . . They provide no ready-made answer to the question "What is history?" '[2] He follows this with the further assertion that:

> The facts, in the first place, do not come to us in pure form but are refracted through the mind of the recorder . . . We thus have to concern ourselves as much with the historians as with their history . . . and search for an objective interpretation and be able to recognise a subjective one.[3]

The views held by the historians of nursing give substance to Carr's observations, for, though treating of the same events and issues, they offer opposing interpretations of their meaning. In an attempt to understand and explain these divergences, alternative evidence will be examined – of the kind that supports the historians' claims, and of the kind that refutes them. This variety of evidence as to what constitutes a proper nurse supplies the grounds of argument for this chapter, which aims to demonstrate ultimately the complex interrelationship that exists between the historian and the events and issues he records.

The Popular Historians' Account of Nineteenth-century Nursing

The first explicit popular histories of what was called 'modern nursing' were published in 1897, on the occasion of Queen Victoria's Jubilee, in the *Nursing Record and Hospital World* and the *British Medical Journal*, and they are taken here as representing the nursing and medical viewpoints of the time. Miss Breay, the author of the *Nursing Record* history, writes:

> Sixty years ago [i.e. 1837] when the Queen ascended the throne, there was neither skilled nursing nor trained nurses as we at the

present day understand these terms. The type of woman who devoted herself to attendance upon the sick because she was fit for nothing else, has been depicted for us by the novelists of that day, in a manner which, even if exaggerated, was recognised at that time to be deserved, and sufficiently scathing to prove that the nurse of the day was not only ignorant, but dangerous to the sick upon whom she was supposed to attend. The immortal character of Sarah Gamp was sufficient to stamp the 'Nurse', during the first third of this century, as a person who disgraced one of the noblest callings to which womankind can devote themselves.[4]

Miss Breay sees private nursing as the root of all other departments of nursing — hospital, workhouse, army, district nursing. Under its heading she writes:

It was three years after the accession of Queen Victoria that Elizabeth Fry, who must always be looked upon as the real pioneer of nursing in this country, recognised the necessity for providing more skilled and trustworthy attendants for the sick of the richer classes; and in order to carry this into effect that most benevolent and far-sighted woman inaugurated the Institution of Nursing Sisters. Mrs Fry's idea evidently was to provide women of character and efficiency. The workers of that day are represented as so hard and cruel that the very name of 'Nurse' was held in horror and contempt, and she probably went as far as the circumstances of the time permitted when she provided for each Nursing Sister to attend at a general hospital for certain hours each day and for a period of a few months, this being recognised as a system of training in advance of anything then existent. The usefulness and trustworthiness of these pioneer Private Nurses led to the formation of a scheme in connection with St. John's House for the better nursing of hospital patients, which, in its turn developed into a further provision of private nurses for the sick of the richer classes. This was inaugurated in 1848 and in succeeding years, one institution after another commenced to supply trustworthy and well-trained nurses for work in private houses. It is interesting and important to observe, therefore, that Private Nursing must be regarded as the Pioneer department of the Profession, and that this, in fact, was called into existence chiefly to meet the demand for careful attendance upon the sick in private houses.[5]

She begins her account of the history of the department of hospital nursing with this ascription: 'The work of St. John's House in training probationers at various Metropolitan hospitals commenced about the year 1848, and to this great religious foundation must therefore be ascribed, the credit of initiating the modern system.'[6] But she goes on to ascribe the proper foundation of the modern system of hospital nursing to Florence Nightingale, though on grounds which differ from those upon which Elizabeth Fry's status as pioneer is established:

> But the establishment of the Nightingale Fund at St. Thomas' Hospital, and especially the work of Miss Nightingale in laying down the foundation principles on which nursing should be conducted, and the relations which should exist between the nursing staff and other hospital workers, must always cause Miss Nightingale to be regarded as the Chief Pioneer of modern hospital nursing in this country.[7]

The medical history, too, gives an account of a change from unskilled and untrustworthy nurses to a kind that were useful and efficient, but we shall see that doctors were less satisfied with the extent and outcome of the remedy than was Miss Breay. The medical historian also claims that the change from Sarah Gamp to the modern nurse has been accomplished within the last sixty years and represents 'a marvellous development and growth' almost synchronous with the reign of Queen Victoria, and that the causes of the development were philanthropic, religious and social. The philanthropic causes ultimately lead to the figure of Mrs Fry, who is viewed as the founder of nursing:

> Her work led her among all forms of suffering and she was moved to make some attempt at organised nursing of the sick poor in London; hitherto the sick had been in the hands of the unprincipled and irresponsible attendants so graphically described by Charles Dickens. The Dowager Queen Adelaide and the Bishop of London joined hands in this laudable effort and the Protestant Nursing Sisters began their work in Whitechapel in 1840. This was the first Nursing Institution and marks the origin of that movement which attained to such proportions in that time; it started from that Quaker lady whose name has hitherto been almost exclusively claimed by the prisoners, but she must now be accepted as the founder of sick nursing.[8]

The religious causes of nursing are linked in this history to the philanthropic causes by their contemporaneity. It continues:

> At the same time, that Revival in the Church, generally known as the Oxford Movement, was awakening in the hearts of earnest women the desire for definite religious work; this wish found its fulfilment for many in the English Sisterhoods, and, for those to whom the severe and dedicated life of the religious was not possible, in a life devoted to the care of nursing of the sick. As soon as the pioneers had demonstrated the possibility of a woman working in the wards of a hospital and yet retaining her womanliness and modesty, such women turned to nursing the poor in hospitals.[9]

Other social causes were seen as accompanying the philanthropic and religious ones:

> In enumerating the religious and social influences at work among women, we must not forget that in the medical profession there was arising a demand for a higher class of women to tend at the bedside. . . For in the 1830's, there was a stir all along the line of the medical profession, prompted by investigations into the conditions under which the sick were treated and into the circumstances surrounding the wounded on the field of battle. The object lessons . . . were pointing the moral that there was a grievous waste of human life from causes which were within the control of man. . . The physician at the bedside and the surgeon in the operating theatre had the conviction forced upon them that if they were to do the best possible for their patients, they wanted hands, gentle, skilful, and sympathetic, which would work with them and for them at the bedside. In other words, the old hospital methods, which had accepted any rough, incapable, and sometimes disreputable female as an attendant on the sick, were found to be insufficient both from the scientific and humanitarian point of view, and the leading members of the medical profession were taking counsel with the leading philanthropists in search of a remedy.[10]

The *British Medical Journal* continues its history by interweaving many famous themes:

> Charles Dickens' graphic portraiture of the nurse of 1848 gave that rude awakening to the national self-respect which was required to

arouse it into action, but it needed a sharper shock before the lethargy of the public conscience was completely overcome. That shock was administered when the sad tales of the sufferings of our soldiers and sailors in the Russian War reached these shores, and it was with a thrill of satisfaction that the nation heard that Florence Nightingale and a band of trained nurses and ladies had left to nurse in the field hospitals of the Crimea.[11]

But Miss Nightingale is not accorded the pioneer status of Miss Breay's history. She is seen as:

not unprepared for the great work which was placed in her hands. In 1851 she had availed herself of the course in Kaiserswerth to obtain an insight into sick nursing and hospital management and later she was Superintendent of the Home for Invalid Ladies in Harley Street. Indeed, it is because she had been a diligent student of the public institutions of this and other countries that when the call came she was ready to answer it. When Miss Nightingale went to the Crimea, she was accompanied by eleven nurses from St. John's House, an institution which is with us to the present day. It owed its foundation in 1848 to the combined efforts of Dr. William Bowman of King's College Hospital and the Bishops of London and Lincoln. This gives us the date of the first attempt at hospital reform. Though here and there in the hospitals a few good examples of a womanly nurse were to be found, it was as the exception to women of the type of Betsy Prig. Sir William Bowman was anxious to improve the nursing of King's College Hospital and an arrangement was entered into with the authorities of St. John's House to provide the nurses and to supervise the wards of the hospital. St. Thomas', under Mrs. Wardroper, was the next to follow and for some time these were the only two hospitals of any size which endeavoured to bring about a better state of sick nursing.[12]

This history also claims that this is the first we hear of the systematic training of nurses:

Until now such special knowledge as distinguished either the Protestant or Roman Catholic nurses was 'acquired' either by the light of Nature or by spending two or more hours in the out patient department of a hospital. Some of the Religious Orders still feel a diffidence at submitting to a hospital training, but others have faced the situation

and accepted the fact that nursing must be learned in the only place
where it can be taught − in a hospital.[13]

Here we are given a view of the proper definition of nursing as already
established, and of Florence Nightingale as its student.

The histories now diverge in their view of the outcome of the
remedies thus begun. For Miss Breay, the advent of explicit principles
of nursing conduct and of nursing arrangements was followed by
further desirable developments. She writes in her history:

> The next important step was the adoption of the three-year system
> of training, and this has now been, after a long discussion, and strong
> opposition, practically admitted to be necessary both for the welfare
> of the sick, and for the most satisfactory working of the training
> schools.[14]

In contrast, the medical historian views the introduction of nursing
training as having led to unsatisfactory results:

> As time passed on [he writes] the training of probationers became
> more specialised; from clinical and practical it became to a greater
> extent theoretical. In moderation there could be nothing but praise
> for this system, but there is no doubt that the theoretical side has
> been overdone; the style and method of training being on the same
> lines as those of the medical student, have not proved equally
> suitable to the sick nurse, whose work is essentially practical and
> whose efficiency depends more on skilful handling and observation
> than on acquaintance with the minutiae of physiology or anatomy.
> A bad style of nurse has resulted from this false training and it is on
> the increase.[15]

For Miss Breay, in contrast, not only has the remedy of a systematic
training been seen to be necessary and satisfactory, but it is also the
proper remedy; and as the proper remedy, it is therefore the proper
foundation for the future development of nursing:

> The authorities of the Training Schools for Nurses are clearly
> realising that for the sake of the inmates of their hospitals, as well as
> for the welfare of the sick of the richer classes, by whose contribu-
> tions the hospitals are supported, it is essential that the education of
> nurses must be conducted upon more systematic and more thorough

principles than have hitherto been the case. The effect of this upon the personnel of the Nursing Profession must in future be very great for the obvious reason that a higher standard of general education will almost necessarily be required from those who purpose to become nurses; while, on the other hand the greater expense to hospitals of the training and board of such probationers, will almost inevitably result in probationers becoming more and more regarded as pupils and less and less treated as servants of the Institution.[16]

All that remains to complete the history of the development of nursing is that:

the nineteenth century, which has witnessed the rise of nursing as a profession should not end without the full accomplishment being reached of this great work, in the foundation of the calling on a secure and settled basis, and the final development of nursing into a Profession recognised and regulated by the State.[17]

The medical historian takes a very different view of the course of nineteenth-century nursing:

To those who have followed the history of the nursing movement it will be evident that, like all great movements, it was begun by individuals, then it was taken up by associated workers, who undertook the nursing of the sick in their own homes, then it penetrated into the hospitals, from which time it began to take rank as a *skilled* profession and attracted to itself large numbers of women of culture, position and education; at that point we now stand. What is still lacking is organisation. The question of Registration has yet to be fought out; but the time has by no means come when legislation can step in to give effect to some one of the many theories which cluster round the scheme. Nurses are not at one on the necessity for Registration and it is unprofitable to discuss methods until the principle is agreed on. (emphasis in original)[18]

These histories of nursing take account of the same events and the same issues, within the same time period between 1837 and 1897. The events are comprised of the work of Elizabeth Fry, the founding of the Institute of Nursing Sisters in 1840 and of St John's House in 1848, of Florence Nightingale's work in the Crimea and the training school founded from the national subscription to her and attached to St Thomas' Hospital in 1861. The issues concern the character of hospital nurses, the desire to stamp out 'Sarah Gamp' and people the occupation with educated women, the nature and purpose of nurse training and the principles upon which the occupation shall become unified and gain a public identity. But, though the events and the issues dealt with are identical, I shall show that they are interpreted and related in each history in a way that exhibits opposing views of what the character and status of nursing was, is and ought to be. I shall also relate these differences to the difference in the pioneer status that each historian accords to Elizabeth Fry and Florence Nightingale, showing that each ascription fits each historian's respective views of hospital nursing.

Miss Breay claims that Elizabeth Fry must always be looked upon as the 'real pioneer' of nursing, for she set out to provide useful and trustworthy nurses for the sick in their homes. She recruited women of character and sent them to general hospitals for about two hours each day for a period of a few months, and there they observed the practice of nursing that was current. The work of her institutes, carried on outside hospitals, incorporated two notions: the notion of selective recruitment and the notion that nursing was something for which a woman required explicit preparation. But though, in Miss Breay's view, the character of hospital nurses was a disgrace and an evil which Mrs Fry recognised, Mrs Fry did not seek to reform them. Rather did her sisters obtain an understanding of nursing among them: 'It was not an easy task which Mrs. Fry undertook' (Miss Breay writes) 'for the workers of that day were so hard and cruel that the very name of "nurse" was held in horror and contempt.'[19]

It would be difficult to begin a history of nursing in Miss Breay's terms of great reforms by according status to that which required reform. Elizabeth Fry did not seek to reform hospital nursing, but to learn from its established practice. She is ascribed the status of real pioneer of nursing because she established a standard for the work that she carried on in private homes, and private nursing, in Miss Breay's view, is the root of all departments of British nursing.

In this history, the 'chief pioneer of modern hospital nursing' is Florence Nightingale, and I shall show how this ascribed status is related to Miss Breay's view of what constitutes a proper definition of hospital nursing.

The new system of nurse training at St Thomas' Hospital was inaugurated in 1861. We are not given a detailed account of the arrangements, and learn only that Florence Nightingale's pioneer work was in the establishment of principles, not only of the conduct of nursing, but also of the relationship that should obtain between nurses and other hospital workers. It is these principles that Miss Breay regards as the ones that are fundamental to all subsequent and future developments in hospital nursing. They incorporate arrangements that would transform the status of hospital nurses from that of servant of the hospital to educated pupil, if only by the financial expenditure entailed.

After enumerating the steps that nursing took after 1861 — the introduction of a three-year system of training, preliminary training schools and hospital examinations, certificates and badges — Miss Breay builds her case for state legitimation of the status of nursing as it then stands. The first principles of the modern system, of training and educating women who have been selectively recruited, form the foundation of these later elaborations and, altogether, they are seen by her as the characteristics of a profession. She asserts that 'it is upon the principle of Profession that the public identity of nursing should be settled'.[20]

Miss Breay is writing from the viewpoint of what she calls the 'modern system', which is what she saw as obtaining in 1897. Discussion of the matter of state registration was held publicly, and it consisted of elaborations of the principles laid down in 1861 at St Thomas' Hospital. Florence Nightingale is accorded status as the pioneer of those principles which, importantly, supplanted the established definitions of nursing and which were also of a kind that could lead eventually to a separate public identity. Such changes could not have followed from Elizabeth Fry who, rather, drew upon the definitions and practices that were already established in the hospitals of the day.

The medical view of nursing history expresses a different opinion of the remedies by which 'Sarah Gamp' has been supplanted. It regards Elizabeth Fry as the founder of nursing on the grounds of the work that she accomplished outside hospitals. When these new types of women enter hospitals to nurse, it is through the philanthropic nursing institutes and the religious sisterhoods that formed in the context of the Oxford Movement, in emulation of the religious communities that existed on the Continent; and what is important when women become nurses in hospitals is that they retain their womanliness, rather than that they have introduced new knowledge and new nursing practice. It is medical knowledge, and its changing understanding of the role of the immediate environment and of the

practices that constituted the treatment of the patient, that is the cause
of a change in the character of hospital nursing:

> if they were to do the best possible for their patients, they wanted
> hands, gentle, skilful, and sympathetic, which would work with
> them and for them at the bedside. In other words, the old hospital
> methods, which had accepted any rough, incapable, and sometimes
> disreputable female as an attendant on the sick, were found to be
> insufficient.

This history dates the 'first attempt at hospital reform' at 1848,
when St John's House Sisterhood first entered King's College Hospital
to take over the nursing of the hospital at the request of Sir William
Bowman, a senior member of the medical staff. The term 'hospital
reform' is followed immediately by a discussion of the womanly
character now required of nurses, and the claim is made that

> this is the first we hear of the systematic training of nurses. Until
> now such special knowledge as distinguished either the Protestant
> or Roman Catholic nurses was 'acquired' either by the light of
> Nature or by spending two or more hours in the out patient
> department of a hospital. Some of the Religious Orders still feel a
> diffidence at submitting to a hospital training, but others have faced
> the situation and accepted the fact that nursing must be learned in
> the only place where it can be taught – in a hospital.

The right kind of womanly character has been obtained, in this view, to
carry out the nursing that has been defined and is being re-defined by
doctors.

We can now begin to sketch an account of what the medical historian
thought that nineteenth-century nursing was and ought to be. The
reforms in the early part of the period were, as for the nursing historian,
reforms of the moral character of nurses – gentle, sympathetic hands
were required to replace rough and incapable hands. But what did
doctors mean by 'skilful hands'? I argue, from the evidence of this
particular history, that doctors wanted a training which would retain
the status of nursing as it was already established – as a set of practices
deriving mainly from medical knowledge, and not as the set of principles
introduced into hospitals through the Nightingale Fund at St Thomas'.

The medical view of the introduction of nurses from the St John's
Sisterhood to King's College Hospital was that it was due, as we have
seen, to a request for it by a senior member of the medical staff, and
that these nurses, although representing a reform of character, were

required to practise nursing as it was already understood by doctors. This 'first attempt at hospital reform' produced 'womanly nurses' who had before this been 'the exception to women of the type of Betsy Prig'. St Thomas' Hospital was next to follow this example and, the argument runs, for some time these were the only two hospitals of any size which endeavoured to bring about a better state of sick nursing. The history claims these events as 'the first we hear of the systematic training of nurses' and as preceding Florence Nightingale's departure to the Crimea; her influence and actions upon her return are regarded as merely the extension of existing principles. She cannot, therefore, be regarded as the founder of a system of nursing viewed as already in existence.

We have seen that Miss Breay upheld the kind of view of hospital nursing that conceived of it not as a set of practices with which a woman could become 'familiarised' in hospital wards, but as entailing new principles, the study and practice of which required new institutional arrangements. The status of hospital nursing was re-defined in them and Miss Breay claimed that they constituted the structure of a complete occupational identity. By contrast, the medical view of these conceptions was that: 'As time passed on the training of probationers became more specialised; from clinical and practical it became to a greater extent theoretical . . . and a bad style of nurse has resulted from this false training.'[23] In this historian's detailed view of the difference between the training of a medical student and the training of a nurse:

> Anything which approximates the training of a nurse to that of a medical student is to be avoided. A thorough acquaintance with the structure of the body and of the various influences to which it is subject is the necessary equipment for a doctor; for the nurse, a knowledge of the laws of life and health, of the functions of the various organs of the body and the outlines of its anatomy would fit her for an intelligent performance of her duties, and leave her ample leisure to make herself proficient in those bedside duties on which depend the comfort and well-being of the patient.[24]

Unlike Miss Breay, who sees 'Profession' as being the settled principle of the state registration of nurses, the medical view is that 'the question of central control and the theories on which it shall be based are unsolved'.[25]

We see that, when nineteenth-century doctors talked of nursing as a 'skilled profession', it was in terms which accepted changes in the character of nurses but which rejected those changes in their status and their work which did not stem from a medical definition of nursing — as a set of practices, deriving mainly from medical knowledge but also comprising a metaphysics, termed 'the laws of life and health', and the unspecified duties involved in attending to the daily comfort and well-being of patients.

The Status of Popular History

We have in these two popular histories opposing views of what nursing was, is and ought to be. In the nursing view, the old methods have been supplanted by a new system, which is regarded as that upon which occupational identity should properly be based. The medical view agrees that there is a new system, but is unsatisfied with its content and disturbed by the attempt to create from it a unified occupational identity. Both place the events of history and the status of its heroines in a relationship that supports their respective points of view. The facts of nursing history, of what it was and now is, seem thus to be judged and interpreted according to what each historian thinks it ought to be.

Carr does not believe that there exists a hard core of historical facts that are objective and independent of the interpretation of the historian.[26] He argues that the element of interpretation enters into every fact of history, that interpretation plays a necessary part in establishing facts and that no interpretation is wholly objective. But he does not consider that this means that the facts of history are in principle not amenable to objective interpretation and that, therefore, one interpretation is as good as another. For Carr, objectivity in history cannot be an objectivity of facts by themselves; it is an objectivity of relation, of the relation between fact and interpretation of fact, between past, present and future.[27]

So far, I have presented the past of nursing through the account we have of it in two of its popular histories and I have argued that their views have related its past, present and future from the standpoint of what may be regarded as their occupational interests and biases. But it is not from argument alone, but from the standpoint also of alternative evidence, that the status of these histories as objective interpretation must be finally assessed, and in the sections that follow I shall explore that evidence. It is constituted of written records, the authors of which were concerned with the construction, not of nursing history, but of the nursing services of nineteenth-century hospitals. The actualities that are considered, and the discussions that take place about them, relate to the everyday character of hospital nursing, its daily work and its relationship to the wider organisation of the hospital. These records supply evidence of nursing as it was being experienced and ordered in actions that had concrete ends, and it is in these terms that I shall construct a critical account, first of the character of hospital nurses and next of their status in relation to those groups with whom they shared the business of daily life and work.

The Alternative Evidence of Nursing History

The Characteristics of Hospital Nurses

The records of history to be analysed in this section are comprised of views about nursing that were publicly expressed and energetically debated. They appeared in laymen's magazines, medical journals and pamphlets and this is itself a fact of significance, for it helps us identify whose point of view it is that we are exploring. Lay magazines of the nineteenth century were the accepted medium of discourse for the leisured upper class, and for the dissemination of the kind of knowledge that was valued by them. Medical journals were contributed to almost exclusively by doctors, whilst nurses possessed no magazine or journal that was exclusively theirs and, between 1840 and 1870, made practically no contribution to public debate. These observations lead us therefore to characterise the debate about hospital nursing as one that was conducted by philanthropists and doctors. Later in this section I shall show the importance of this point in helping us to trace the source of the reputation that was accorded to hospital nurses.

In *Fraser's Magazine* for May 1848, the writer declares, in an article entitled 'Hospital Nurses as they are and as they ought to be', that:

> it is notorious that the present race of hospital nurses do not come up to the standards of the very ideal of nurses — women of patience, gentleness and self-devotion of the kind of the Sisters of Charity. Mrs. Gamp may be a caricature, but her likeness is very traceable.[28]

The *Medical Times and Gazette* for 1852 writes: '. . . a paid nurse of the old school. We in the Profession well know what that means — a hard-minded, ignorant and lazy woman, who sleeps when she should be awake and is cross when she should be patient.'[29] *Household Words* for 1858 reports:

> London now has a training school for nurses in St. John's House,

whose declared purpose is to improve the qualifications and raise the
character of nurses for the sick by providing for them professional
training together with moral and religious discipline under the care
of a clergyman . . . It has been joined to King's College Hospital in
an effort to supplant Mrs. Gamp with a trained nurse.[30]

In *Once a Week* for December 1859, Harriet Martineau writes:

> How much good nursing have any of us ever seen — wherever there
> are mothers and daughters there will be good nursing as far as it can
> be taught by good sense and affection. But nursing is an art based
> upon science, and the resources of instinct, insufficient in individual
> cases, are as nothing in times of accident and epidemic sickness.
> Meanwhile, to be, to do and to talk 'like an old nurse' means to be
> positive, ignorant and superstitious . . . But the time is at hand, the
> money is in the bank and the plan is under discussion for the training
> of women in the art of nursing.[31]

In the *Cornhill Magazine* for February 1865, a plea is made for a
response to the advertisements for women to train under the
Nightingale Fund:

> for the unemployed educated, or middle class women of the day to
> train as nurses, and readers are assured that the past of nursing has
> nothing to do with the nurses of the present subject . . . The
> traditional monthly nurse and her sister of the sick room — ignorant,
> gossiping, full of mischievous superstition and fancies — has been
> replaced in the last dozen years by just so much progress made as to
> give us a little taste of the comfort of a trained nurse in the anxious
> seasons of life.[32]

From this date onwards 'Sarah Gamp' becomes less a fact to be
observed than a tradition to be remembered, but up to this date this
evidence supports the historians' view of the once disreputable character
of hospital nurses. It does so, as we can see, in the context of the belief
that this must be remedied by selective recruitment and training.
Further, it is largely the evidence of philanthropists, whose claims can be
seen to include also the content of what the popular historians have
called the great reforms in the character of nurses. Yet it does not
constitute all the alternative evidence that is knowable, and I discuss
now the views that were held by those who wanted not reform, but

'improvement', and upon not different but established bases.

In 1857, John South, Senior Surgeon to St Thomas' Hospital, published a pamphlet entitled 'Facts Relating To Hospital Nurses'.[33] This paper is a reply to public accusations about nurses, of the sort that have already been quoted. John South replies that he 'is not disposed to allow that the nursing establishments of our hospitals are insufficient, or that they are likely to be improved by any special institute for the training, sustenance and protection of hospital nurses and attendants'.[34] He then describes what he sees as facts:

> As regards the nurses or ward-maids, these are much in the condition of housemaids and require little teaching beyond that of poultice-making, which is easily acquired, and the enforcement of cleanliness and attention to patients' wants. They need not be of the class of persons required for Sisters, not having such responsibility. I have known but few of these persons who have become competent to promotion to the higher class. But if encouragement by increased remuneration and the certainty of promotion to the well-conducted and the capable were held out, I feel assured that the application for appointment as nurses or ward-servants would not be wanting from women of better station than those we now have.[35]

In Guy's Hospital Reports for 1871 Dr Steele writes of this period around 1859 and of the nursing arrangements that obtained at Guy's Hospital:

> For the more subordinate appointment of nurse, which at the time referred to included not only attendance on the more immediate wants of the sick, but the cleaning and scrubbing of ward floors and of the staircases of the hospital, it was necessary to select from a class of inferior grade to the others. Persons offering themselves for the office were, usually speaking, but little removed from the ordinary class of domestic servants . . . As far as my experience leads me I believe that similar systems existed in all hospitals and as regarded their individual efficiency they were all very much on an equality . . . In the selection of persons for the office of nurse, preference is given to a good class of domestic servants between the ages of 20 and 40 years. After a woman has taken to the work it rarely happens that she leaves it. It sometimes, though rarely, happens that they are discharged for misconduct. Occasional instances of drunkenness occur but the more common and venial faults are

incompatibility of temper, staying out without leave . . . or neglect of some important duty — offences which do not always prove a barrier to their obtaining employment elsewhere.[36]

From these discussions we can construct a view of the nineteenth-century hospital nurse as belonging to a grade the duties and position of which were defined in terms partly of domestic service and partly of very loosely specified nursing tasks deriving mainly from medical theory. 'Patients' immediate wants', to which this type of nurse attended, were not specified. The lengthy hours of work, the payment of a weekly wage, the accommodation in dormitories that Dr Steele regards, in other parts of his article, as an 'improvement', are comparable to the working conditions of nineteenth-century domestic servants in private households. The nursing tasks were those that were easily taught, they were not clearly demarcated from domestic service to the hospital and all aspects of the nurse/ward-maid grade were subject to the immediate supervision and control of the ward sister. If characterisation of early-nineteenth-century hospital nurses is to provide objective history in Carr's sense, then it must take account of these structural features, rather than be constructed from the language of subjective description. 'Sarah Gamp' is a literary character, and is a fact of history just exactly in that way, and it is the use of her as a characterisation of hospital nurses which has to be explained. The evidence just considered presents a view of a state of affairs that, though not satisfactory in the eyes of the writers, Mr South and Dr Steele, is not either described by them as 'the evils of hospital nursing' or as 'an opprobrium'. It remains a matter for further study to discover the reasons why hospital nurses were accorded publicly the reputation of an irresponsible Gamp. I suggest that these reasons may be discovered in the philanthropic movement, which sought to reform hospital nursing by arrangements that were either alien and external to existing arrangements, or else were not implicit in these arrangements. The public debate accords the character of 'Sarah Gamp' to nurses in the context of reforms that consisted of the introduction of the nursing institutes and religious sisterhoods, and, twenty years later, of the introduction into St Thomas' Hospital of what Miss Breay calls 'the modern system'. In contrast, both Mr South and Dr Steele discuss hospital nurses in a context which expresses the view that their training can be accommodated upon existing institutional arrangements, within each hospital as an entity independent of every other in the voluntary system. Like our historians' accounts, these descriptions of what hospital nurses were can be seen to relate to claims of what each thought nurses ought to be. I suggest that the characterisation of the hospital nurse as 'Sarah Gamp' was created at the time to support philanthropic claims for changes that were based on different ideals and different social arrangements from those that obtained, and that it is a reputation rather than a set of facts that has become incorporated into popular nursing history. I shall now examine the evidence of these arrangements and construct from them an account of the status of hospital nurses in the different systems that are encountered – the nursing institutes connected with Mrs Fry, the religious sisterhoods and the system founded at St Thomas' Hospital, which was popularly known as the pioneer of 'the modern system'.

The Status of Hospital Nurses

The Established System.   The term 'status' indicates the rights and obligations of any individual relative to those of others and to the scale of worthwhileness that obtains in the group, whatever it may be. We have seen that the status of hospital nursing in the organisation of early-nineteenth-century hospitals was that of practically the lowest servant of the institution. In this section I shall attempt to trace the change from that status to one of probationer and pupil of the hospital, and show how it was shaped by domestic organisation, both within and without the ward, and by the position of the ward sister as the immediate controller of the daily domestic and nursing work of the ward. I shall also consider the relationship that obtained between the ward sister and the ward physician or surgeon and argue that it was of a kind that exercised constraint upon radical changes in the status and the work of the hospital nurse. It is in terms of these structural features that I identify systems of nursing, and I begin by considering the system which the medical historian considered to be established long before Florence Nightingale embarked for the Crimea.

The nursing system of early-nineteenth-century hospitals comprised the office of matron, the office or grade of sister, and the grade of nurse or ward maid. The term 'office' contrasts with that of 'grade' in that, where 'office' is a defined position of the institution to which rights as well as duties, and a notion of tenure, attached, 'grade' specified duties alone, without rights or expectation of tenure. The system was under the control of the lay administration, which had the ultimate right of engagement to and dismissal from all nursing positions. Internal authority was variously distributed between matron and sister, depending on the size of the institution. All domestic and nursing matters were under the control of the matron but the daily management of the domestic and nursing work of each ward devolved upon the ward sister. But we shall see that the position of ward sister was also kept under close medical control. Evidence that this system generally obtained exists in the *British Medical Journal* of 1880, in which an article on nursing systems, and so entitled, describes the positions and relations of matron/ward sister/nurse under the heading 'Ward Systems, one of three at present in vogue'.[37]

Mr South describes the nursing system at St Thomas' Hospital thus:

For the ordinary service of each ward the nurses are of three kinds, two day nurses and a night nurse or ward-maid as she is more properly designated in Dublin hospitals . . . The control and responsible charge of the ward rests with the 'Sister' or head nurse, and the nurse or 'ward maid' has the menial offices to perform . . . Each sister is provided with a bedroom and sitting room adjoining the ward and one or both opening into it, but the greater part of her day is spent in the ward . . . if she has any serious case on hand she is more frequently up night after night . . . She receives a salary paid quarterly and no rations except beer . . . It would naturally be presumed that the women filling the office of ward sister, and of nurses or ward servants, are not all of the same class . . . The sister has much the same duty imposed on her as a good private nurse. She receives the directions of the physician or surgeon to whose ward she is attached and she reports to the apothecary or house-surgeon in their absence, any circumstances which call for immediate attention. She takes care that the nurse or ward maid does her duty . . . In severe cases she pays more especial attention to the patients which, but for her unremitting care and womanly aid would not attain successful issue . . . Among this superior class the change is not very frequent . . . Of the surgical sisters, two have been sisters for eighteen years, one seventeen years, one has been sister twenty-two years, another fifteen and another twelve years.[38]

The report of the nursing arrangements at Guy's Hospital refers to the same time period as that of Mr South:

In all hospitals it has been found impossible to carry out the work in a satisfactory way without the assistance of other officers to supervise and give manual and effective aid to the nurses while engaged in the performance of their duties. These officers, to whom various designations have been attached, have always been received at this hospital by the name of Sisters; and to circumscribe the duties of the office, as well as to make the holder personally responsible for a selected charge, it appears to have been the custom at all times for each ward to have the benefit of supervision by a separate sister, who, in addition to the care of the sick, should have charge of the ward stores and also be the medium of communication between the patients and the medical staff. It formerly was the practice to select for this office respectable females who, previous to their appointment had experience of household work, been upper servants in private families, or been engaged in the capacity of nursing the sick out of doors, and not unfrequently the post was filled by one of the ordinary nurses whose promotion was merited from length of service and presumed suitability . . . The Sisters received a salary of £50 annually with an additional allowance of milk and beer . . . Since 1859 there has been an addition to their remuneration and a daily ration of bread, and Sisters are furnished with appropriate costume, while their apartments are furnished at hospital expense, where formerly they had to find furniture.[39]

Of St Thomas' Hospital, Mr South reports of the accommodation of the nurses and of their daily duties:

The day nurse or ward maid performs for the ward the usual duties of a housemaid as to cleaning and bedmaking. She also makes and applies the poultices and the like and attends to the wants of patients confined to their beds . . . She comes on duty at six o'clock in the morning and remains till 8 o'clock in the evening, after which she retires to sup and sleep among her fellows in a spacious dormitory specially allotted to them . . . She is under the immediate superintendence and control of the sister who reports her to the matron or steward if she is negligent.[40]

Of Guy's Hospital arrangements, Dr Steele writes:

Among the improvements carried out with the view of promoting the comfort of the nurses not the least important was the provision made many years ago to supply them with good sleeping accommodation with appropriate furniture and requirements. Bearing in mind the unhealthy character of their employment, it was thought advisable to have their sleeping apartments away from the wards and from the old form of ward dormitory.[41]

The hospital nurse, in terms of the social class to which she was regarded as belonging, the accommodation provided for her, the payment she received and the duties she performed, was entirely subordinate to the ward sister. But her status began to change in all four respects. Of St Thomas', Mr South writes:

> Of late years the nurses have been much improved, in their length of stay in the hospital, and in their competence, by the dormitory system; and if encouraged by increased remuneration and the certainty of promotion for the well-conducted and the capable, then the application for appointment as nurses or ward servants would not be wanting from women of better station than we now have.[42]

The Guy's Hospital report by Dr Steele reads:

> Since the period referred to there has been a progressive tendency in this as well as in most hospitals to increase the number of nurses in proportion to the patients, as well as to separate the work of nursing from that of the ordinary domestic, and otherwise to improve the social position of the nurse . . . In order to avoid the abuses so liable to occur from a system of board wages in place of food . . . [peculation from the patients' diets] . . . the nurses are now furnished with every article of food they are likely to require, and a substantial dinner is daily provided for them in an appropriate dining hall apart from the wards, in which they mess in two relays, so that the wards shall not be deprived of their services at this important period of the day.[43]

As part of this progress, day and night nurses were now also treated alike where before there had been differences in their status in terms of payment received and the amount of nursing done relative to domestic work.

But among these changes in the status of hospital nurses was the introduction at this time of the practice of selective recruitment and of probation. Guy's Hospital reports read:

> In the attempts which have been made, and are still being made, for the improvement of nursing, one common object is kept in view by those interested in the success of the experiment, namely, the

selection of a class of woman of good character, and fitted for the work, whether they have or have not had previous experience, and the discovery of the best means to retain them in the service. To test their fitness, and to render them familiar with the duties they are likely to be called upon to perform, it is of first importance that each candidate for the office should undergo a longer or shorter period of probation, in proportion to her capacities.[44]

These new practices, along with the changes in other aspects of the status of the nurse, now approximated her position more closely to that of the ward sister. The work now required persons of similar character to the sister, whom it was worth while to instruct, and the work was now regarded as of sufficient importance to require instruction. Both ward sister and nurse or ward-maid were recruited, not to statuses within an occupation, but to duties within a hospital ward and positions in the hospital. Though there were improvements in the social position of the sister within the hospital, her ward duties could not change, whilst the nurse or ward maid was now, through the separation of domestic from nursing tasks, and the change in the proportion of nurses to patients, becoming more of a nurse than she had formerly been. Yet, in practice, the separation of domestic from nursing work was incomplete, for Guy's Hospital report states that:

Though the work of scrubbing the floors is done by a regular staff of women, supplemented by charwomen who attend at convenient intervals . . . it cannot be said that the result of this division of labour entirely severs the nursing from the subordinate work of scrubbing. It is also somewhat difficult to say how a nurse's time could be fully occupied if she were retained only to administer to the sick, and it is difficult to draw a hard line of demarcation between the supplementary work required in every establishment and the more exclusive duty of nursing.[45]

Of all these aspects of change in the status of the nurse, I consider the most significant to be those discussed latterly — the practice of probation and the notion within it of the teaching of nursing, and the attempt to separate the duties of nurse from the duties of domestic servant. I shall consider the pupillage of nurses, not as an abstract principle, but as it was worked out in the context of the daily management of the ward and its work, and of its supervision by the ward sister. These matters constitute the system of authority and control over the work of nurses that shaped and constrained it, and that, reciprocally, was most modified by the nurse's transition from servant to pupil. I shall discuss next, therefore, some relevant aspects of the office of ward sister. Mr South describes their appointment and probation at St Thomas':

> The sisters, when selected, are not thrust at once into the wards, ignorant and ill-fitted for the responsibilities they assume, to pick up a knowledge of their business as best they can. They are at first taken as supernumeraries, or unattached, into the matron's office, where, by their frequent errands into the wards, and communications with the attached sister, they gradually attain an insight into the duties they will have to undertake; and after a while are sent for short periods into a ward. The probationary sister, when appointed to a ward, must not assume that up to this time her education is complete. She has still much to learn, which can only be attained in the ward, by the kind and patient assistance and guidance of the physician or surgeon to whom she is attached. What sort of attendant she shall be depends, *coeteris paribus*, mainly on him.[46]

We may characterise the pupillage of hospital nurses as practised in wards where domestic, nursing and medical interests were closely interwoven, but where the doctor, through his long-standing relationship with a ward sister who held permanent tenure of office, controlled the status of nursing as a set of practical duties to be defined by him. I shall argue throughout this chapter that the definition of nursing and of its day-to-day control through the ward physician/ward sister relationship is of central significance in considering changes in the status and work of the nurse.

In this section, what Mr South, Dr Steele and other doctors, writing in the medical journals of the time, take to be the established system of nursing has been discussed. In the next section I shall explore the ways in which the systems of nursing institutes, of religious sisterhoods and of training founded at St Thomas' Hospital affected the source of control and definition of nursing that has been asserted to be the most significant factor in the transition of hospital nurses from the status of servant to pupil. I shall argue that what the nursing historian of the *Nursing Record and Hospital World* regards as a proper foundation of nursing can be seen to be a system in which a nurse's work is defined and taught not only within the ward but from an authority that operates outside it, and with reference, not to the nurse only as performer of ward duties and thereby as servant of the hospital, but to the nurse as pupil.

The Institute of Nursing Sisters 1840.   Both the Guy's and St Thomas' Hospital surgeons report their view of the nursing arrangements of the Institute of Nursing Sisters, founded by Mrs Fry in 1840. Dr Steele reports:

> Many societies which have been originated for the supply of nurses to the sick have gladly availed themselves of the opportunity allowed them at Guy's Hospital for instructing their probationers in the art. Among those may be mentioned the Nursing Sisters Institution, established by the celebrated Mrs. Fry in 1840, which has an active staff of nearly 100 women constantly engaged in attention on the sick in private houses . . . There are usually two probationers from the institution at work in the hospital, where they remain for a period of two months, apportioning their time betwixt the medical, surgical and obstetric wards, so that on average 12 women receive the benefit of instruction during the year.[47]

Mr South states:

> The Institution of Nursing Sisters, founded by the exertions of the late Mrs. Fry in 1840, proposes only to prepare and provide nurses . . . The nursing sisters under instruction have enjoyed the large opportunities for practical knowledge afforded them by Guy's Hospital from the first foundation of the Institution in 1840; and within the last five or six years (from 1851) they have been also received at St. Thomas', where we have constantly two or three of them. I must confess that when they first came I was not all in favour of the arrangement, as I feared inconvenience would arise from interference with the ward duties, which I consider it is always the duty of the medical officer to promote; but my fears on this point have entirely passed away. The women are attentive and observant . . . and on the best possible terms with the sisters of the wards. When considered qualified, they return to the Institution house where they continue under the control of the lady superintendent, until appointed as required and applied for.[48]

Both these views hold that the existing arrangements for nursing in their hospitals do not merely define what must be learned by those who wish to nurse, but are arrangements by which their own nurses are successfully made. Mr South comments of his description of the facts of nursing that 'I think I have shown that we have within our hospitals all the apparatus for making the best sisters and our experience shows that we do make them'.[49] Of Guy's Hospital, the report reads: 'The advantages and facilities afforded by the hospital for practical instruction, and so largely availed of for the purposes of a medical school, renders it also an excellent training institution for nurses.'[50] Neither did the Nursing Institute founded by Mrs Fry seek to usurp this system. It sought to learn from it, and further, in order to supply nurses privately and outside hospitals, in the homes of rich or poor.

The popular historians of nursing have accorded pioneer status to Mrs Fry and the principles adopted by her of selective recruitment and of training. But we cannot see these events as differing, except in their form, from the practice of selecting and training hospital sisters. This practice long preceded its extension to the grade of nurse in the 1850s and 1860s, but Mrs Fry's nurses were likewise called nursing sisters and therefore must be compared with their counterparts in the hospitals of the time. Further, Mrs Fry's Institute was an institute of philanthropy, as were the voluntary hospitals, in which the sisters were paid. Dr South writes that 'the outgoings of the Institute were: salaries of sisters, £1,769 12s. 6d',[51] amongst other items. The arrangements of the Institute of Nursing Sisters founded by Mrs Fry cannot so far be proven as the founding arrangements of nursing.[52]

The nursing historians have claimed that St John's House Sisterhood 'initiated the modern system' – this is Miss Breay's claim – and represented 'the first attempt at hospital reform' – this is the medical historian's claim. In order to assess these claims, I shall examine next the advent of St John's House nurses and sisters at King's College Hospital and the status of hospital nursing within this system, not with reference to changes in the type of payment and accommodation that they received, but in terms of the probation of nurses in wards that were controlled by ward sisters in the established arrangements already described.

St John's House Sisterhood 1848. In the records of the St John's House archives we may read that its sisterhood had its own council of management, expressing both medical and episcopal sanction in the composition of this council of eminent medical staff from King's College Hospital and of bishops. Its object was to recruit women to membership of itself as a community of sisters who would train nurses for the sick. It instituted the office of lady superintendent which, together with its title, was merged for technical reasons with the office of matron of the hospital, the grade of sister, whose work was gratuitous, and the grade of nurse, a person who was trained to her work. At the bottom of these grades was the probationer, a person who was training for the grade and title of nurse. Sisters were ladies of birth and performed their duties as an act of religious commitment and service to the sisterhood. Nurses and probationers were paid, but were selectively recruited according to standards that were comparable to the grade of sister, except in the matter of what was seen as their social class. All candidates to all grades had to furnish certificates of baptism into the Church of England and of character. In the archives a record is to be found of a 'Statement by the Lady Superintendent to Lord Hatherley, of the Council of St. John's House'. In this statement we read:

> It may be well to state in what respects our system of nursing differs from that usually employed at King's College Hospital . . . First, in all the women engaged being Church women of perfectly respectable character, as far as can be ascertained by careful investigation beforehand; secondly, in their being trained under ladies [nursing sisters] who know a nurse's work thoroughly, and who seek to infuse a high tone among those learning it. Then, in their having a full year's training before they are admitted to be 'nurses'. Next, in there not being a separate and lower grade of persons taken for assistant nurses, probationers and night nurses – the latter the most important of any – but all work, from the first step to the highest, in their turn and are stimulated by the certainty that they will earn promotion by care and good conduct. It follows, therefore, that every year a certain number become nurses, and that their place is taken by newcomers . . . Thus a constant supply of good workers is maintained.[53]

It can be seen that a hierarchy of statuses has been established in a way that matches the grades of work that were required to be carried on in hospital wards, and it is structured and organised in terms of a career. Hospital nursing, from the sister to the night nurse, now represents a scale of worthwhileness to which each grade of nurse and of work on the ward belongs. In the established system of nursing that was discussed in the previous section, the nurse, even with the status of pupil, was valued as a servant of the hospital. Dr Steel regarded probation and pupillage as 'an arrangement which will probably have the effect ultimately of retaining the women longer in the service of the hospital'.[54] St John's House, too, was concerned to keep up a supply of workers, but with the possibility for these workers of gaining the rewards of higher status in the higher grades of the sisterhood. In the established system, the rights of the probationer nurse were distributed in terms that referred ultimately to her obligations of service to the hospital in a permanently subordinate status to that of the ward sister. St John's House system distributed rights to the probationer on different terms. Not only was she a candidate for higher status in structural terms, she was also expressly valued as an individual and a member of a community of sisters equally with its other members. The lady superintendent writes:

> It further follows from the St. John's House system, that every nurse is herself an object of personal solicitude to the Superior, who endeavours to allot to each the work for which she is best fitted . . . A St. John's House nurse is not regarded by her superiors as a drudge, who is to be worked for the convenience of others until she can work no longer and then cast aside as useless.[55]

To characterise and practise hospital nursing duties in these terms, in which all levels of ward work are seen as a responsibility for which a nurse is progressively and systematically trained, is to separate them from the characteristics and practice of domestic work as this was understood at the time. In the management of the domestic organisation of the hospital exclusively by the St John's House Sisterhood, the definition of nursing as an occupation exclusive of domestic service to the hospital was further created and maintained. But this control by St John's House of all the domestic affairs of King's College Hospital did not entail a practical separation between nursing and domestic duties. In the daily life of the ward, the nurse continued to perform cleaning duties. However, the status of these duties was itself raised to that of duties that were now regarded as integral to nursing, for they were now defined in terms that approximated to the language of science. Writing in the period of the early 1870s, the lady superintendent claims:

> In this arrangement, St. John's House was in advance of its time, but the auxiliary departments of the hospital (the departments of the kitchen, and of linen, and bedding supplies) are now regarded as forming an integral part of nursing as scientifically understood.[56]

The nursing system of St John's House thus not only controlled the domestic work of the hospital but re-defined it:

> Inasmuch, then, in conducing to the recovery of the sick, the efficiency and good quality of medical or surgical attendance — it would seem that, after securing good physicians and surgeons, the next duty of Hospital authorities is to secure good nurses and to place them in circumstances which enable them to fulfil their engagements.[57]

The 'circumstances' were the auxiliary departments of the hospital, the control of which in this system flowed from the lady superintendent who also controlled the organisation of nursing; thus, both departments of hospital work were controlled independently of the lay administration. The domestic work was conceived of in the St John's House nursing system as having reference to what were regarded as physical conditions integral to the treatment of the sick, and these physical conditions were, in turn, medically prescribed:

> A nurse is responsible [the lady superintendent writes in her 'Statement'] for the maintenance of all the physical conditions which are medically prescribed — that is to say, for the cleanliness and purity of her ward, and of the bedding, dressings, and persons of the sick, for proper ventilation, and the regulation of temperature . . . She cannot maintain physical conditions if . . . insufficiently supplied with fuel and if the requisite changes of bedding are not accessible to her; or if, when supplied, they are found unsuitable for the purposes for which they were desired.[58]

But though the nursing system of St John's House imported radically different structural arrangements into King's College Hospital, it did not create a written theory of nursing. All instruction was practical and flowed from arrangements that were, as in the established system of nursing, internal to the ward and which reflected the relationship between ward physician or surgeon and ward sister that already obtained. The ward sister continued to hold permanent tenure of office and carried out bedside programmes of nursing that were formulated by doctors and communicated to her alone — directly and verbally. The only written formulations of bedside nursing were contained in a four-page pamphlet issued by St John's House authorities, entitled 'Hints for Nurses'. In this pamphlet, nursing knowledge regarding the observation of patients is loosely formulated and carries rather more moral than scientific instruction in nursing:

> The sentinel on duty has to keep watch and protect human life against any sudden assault, and warn the garrison . . . of the approach of danger . . . Medical treatment can be accomplished only by the greatest watchfulness and care in the use of remedies . . .[59]

The training of the ladies as ward sisters was required to be, in order for them to gain this appointment, very much a personal affair, if they were trained at all. I argue, from this evidence, that nursing was defined as a set of practical duties, in this system as in the established systems of nineteenth-century hospitals, to be formulated by doctors and communicated to ward sisters in the context of a long-standing relationship based upon the permanent tenure of both in their respective office, which centred on the hospital ward. The teaching of the probationer comprised practical instruction from the sister in the sphere of the ward, from which the probationer came and went in the course of instruction in the nursing treatment of various types of disease. There existed no source of nursing knowledge that was external to the sphere of the ward. In this way, the status of hospital nursing as a set of practical duties pertaining to hospital wards was unchanged, as was its status as subordinate in this respect to medical control.

We can agree with our medical historian that the St John's House system represented the 'first attempt at hospital reform' if we add the above qualification.

St Thomas' Hospital 1861.   In this final part I shall consider the system of training hospital nurses that was inaugurated at St Thomas' Hospital in 1861, and show that it established the status of the hospital nurse as pupil not only in principle but, importantly, in practice. I argue that this was accomplished by arrangements that removed the control of ward nursing duties from the office and person of ward sister to a sphere that was external to the ward, thus modifying the hitherto exclusive control of the ward sister in allocating ward duties to the pupil nurse.

In his pamphlet entitled 'Suggestions for Improving the Management of the Nursing Department of Large Hospitals',[60] published in 1867, Henry Bonham-Carter, secretary to the fund publicly subscribed to Florence Nightingale on her return from the Crimea and used to finance

the system of nurse training at St Thomas' Hospital, asserts that the
principle of nurse training as essential for nurses is assumed by all his
remarks on hospital nursing; and he argues:

> That in most of our large hospitals is to be found a considerable
> number of skilled nurses is to be admitted, but the system has not
> been successful because nursing has not been considered an art to be
> taught and therefore no provisions have been made for teaching it.
> The end to be gained in any attempt to reform the prevailing system
> of hospital nursing is to substitute trained for untrained nurses.[61]

Mr Bonham-Carter elaborates the conception of a nurse's training that is
to be adopted at St Thomas': 'Good nursing does not grow of itself; it is
the result of study, training, teaching and practice, ending in sound
tradition, which can be transferred elsewhere.'[62] To put this conception
of nursing into practice, the period of training for an admitted
probationer was one year. Her training was defined in terms of service
as 'Assistant Nurse in the wards of the hospital', and the probationer's
work was formulated, not in terms of a new theory of nursing, but in
terms of 'Ward Duties'. On entry to the hospital, each probationer nurse
was supplied with a written list entitled 'Duties of the probationer
under the Nightingale Fund'. Though in this way nursing was specified
as a set of ward practices, nevertheless these were set down in writing,
and given to the probationer before she reached the ward. This is
reminiscent of St John's House 'Hints for Nurses', but whilst the latter
can be seen as a handbook of mere advice to probationers, the St
Thomas' booklet was given a formal status in their training. To ensure
that these duties were carried into practice, both probationer and ward
sister were supplied with books in which the probationer's practical
competence was recorded. In Mr Bonham-Carter's pamphlet, we read:

> To ensure efficiency, each Ward 'Sister' is supplied with a Book,
> which corresponds generally with the List of Duties given to the
> Probationer on her entrance. The columns in the Ward Sister's Book
> are filled up once a week with suitable marks.[63]

In this way, the nurse's work seems defined as a set of practices to
be controlled by the ward sister and constituting service to the hospital.
But these books were examined monthly in matron's office, and were
seen by matron as the written evidence that the principles of training
and the status of pupil or probationer had been carried into practice.

This evidence was, further, examined annually by the committee of the Nightingale Fund which controlled the financial expenditure of the nurse's training, and was not in any respect subject to the scrutiny of the hospital's lay management. A nurse's probation was thus controlled from outside the ward as fulfilment of the principles of probation, as well as within the ward in fulfilment of the nurse's obligations of service to the hospital.

The status of ward sister as supervisor and teacher of nurses in the ward was maintained and there is evidence that those recruited into the system at St Thomas', unlike the sisters recruited to St John's House, were required to be trained. Mr Bonham-Carter writes: 'For effective supervision in the Nursing Department, the "Sisters" or Chief Nurses of the Wards must have been properly trained for the work.'[64] Later on, we read that: '. . . upon the Sisters should depend chiefly the instruction and training of the Under Nurses . . . This point is of great importance.'[65]

It can be seen from these precepts for the management of nurse training that elements of the control of the daily life and work of nurses on the wards remained in the office of ward sister and, if trained, she would have received this training under the established system that has been discussed. But in the institution of the sister's book and the daily diary of bedside nursing that probationers were later expected to maintain, the control of the teaching of probationers passed outside the ward. The ward sister's book, and its examination monthly in matron's office, also limited the freedom of the ward sister to allocate ward duties to the probationer in any arbitrary fashion, as she was able to do in the established system. By these means, I argue, the status of probationer was secured in practice. Nor could the status of the hospital nurse as pupil of the hospital be undermined by the matron, for in this nursing system it was proposed to separate the office of matron and the domestic and household duties which attached to the office from the new status of superintendent of nurses:

Under the present system in most of our hospitals [Mr Bonham-Carter writes] the Matron is the nominal chief of the Nursing Department. Her principal duties are, however, considered to be those of housekeeping. She is almost invariably selected for her qualifications in this respect. It rarely if ever happens that she has had any previous knowledge of the duties of nursing . . . The arrangement of any large hospital must be such that either the housekeeping duties are altogether separated from those of the

Superintendent of Nurses, or . . . that the Matron or Superintendent
shall have an Assistant as Housekeeper.[66]

On a hospital ward the separation of domestic duties and nursing duties
is not merely a matter of principle: it is a problem of actual arrangements. We may conjecture that in practice the probationer continued to
carry out domestic duties in the ward, in spite of radical re-arrangements
of the hospital's nursing and domestic control, for in the 'List of Duties'
given to her on entry to training we see a duty to 'keep the ward fresh
by day and by night' that, though referring to ventilation, is yet
susceptible to varying interpretation.

Miss Breay has claimed that Florence Nightingale is to be regarded as
the 'chief pioneer' of hospital nursing, in laying down the foundations
upon which nursing should be conducted and the relations which should
exist between nurses and other hospital staff. I argue that it is not the
definition of nursing as a set of practices that has changed, but rather
the source of control of those practices in different social arrangements
from those obtaining in the established system of nursing. The ward
sister's book at St Thomas' Hospital represents the first written record
of a nurse's practical competence, and it is the elaboration of this
'examination' of the nurse as pupil, and of arrangements for examination that were external to the ward, that Miss Breay sees as the
constitution of a proper conception and control of nursing. The medical
historian, as we have seen, rejected these arrangements as leading to 'a
bad style of nurse', whose knowledge 'would not be sufficiently distinct
from that of the medical student'.

Both historians of nursing have treated the principles of the selective
recruitment and training of nurses as having been introduced into
hospitals, and as the principles upon which the progress of nursing is
based. In this chapter I have shown that features of those principles
obtained in different forms and in varying degrees in all the systems
that have been considered. But the status of hospital nurse, I have
argued, was a status that was constrained in practice by the control
exercised over the daily duties of the ward by the ward sister. Further,
the ward sister obtained her knowledge of nursing by verbal communication with the doctor, and could control the amount of this
knowledge that was passed on to the nurse. In this way, the nurse's
status as pupil of nursing was, in practice, an arbitrary arrangement and
was a status that could even be undermined. I have attempted to show
that, in the St Thomas' Hospital system, the control of the ward sister
over the practice of nursing in the ward, and the constraint exercised

upon the status of the nurse as pupil, was radically modified by the introduction of arrangements which established this control from outside the ward.

Summary

In the first section of this chapter I argued that nursing history has been presented to us by its nursing and medical authors in a way that reflects their occupational interests. In subsequent sections I have tried to show the facts concerning hospital nursing as these were recorded by writers whose concern was to supply nursing services to hospitals. Each of these writers, like the historians, has expressed his view of what nursing ought to be, and we may argue, therefore, that we still do not possess an objective history of nursing. The account of nursing which has been constructed from these views recognises the interests of each writer and makes no judgement about which of the systems considered should be regarded as exhibiting the 'proper' principles and arrangements of nursing. Rather it demonstrates the everyday conduct of nursing upon which each writer has built his view of what principles and arrangements should be instituted. But it is from the everyday practice of nursing, of its working arrangements in relation to itself and to the wider organisation of the hospital, that I maintain that a history of nursing, in E. H. Carr's sense, should be built. Carr's sense of objective history requires an objectivity of relationship between past, present and future, and between observer and observed. I have tried to accomplish this objectivity by analysing the relationship between the everyday facts of nineteenth-century hospital nursing and the views about those facts that are available to us in a variety of written records of history.

Notes

1. The work on which this chapter is based was originally financed by a Fellowship from the Scottish Home and Health Department.
2. E. H. Carr, *What is History?* (Penguin Books, Harmondsworth, 1970), p. 19.
3. Ibid., p. 22ff.
4. Margaret Breay, 'Nursing in the Victorian Era', *Nursing Record and Hospital World* (19 June 1897), pp. 493–502.
5. Ibid., pp. 493–4.
6. Ibid., p. 494.
7. Ibid., p. 496.
8. 'The Nursing of the Sick Under Queen Victoria', *British Medical Journal,*

vol. 1 (19 June 1897), pp. 1644–8. No author is given for this article.
    9. Ibid., p. 1645.
    10. Ibid., pp. 1645–6.
    11. Ibid., p. 1646.
    12. Ibid., p. 1646.
    13. Ibid., p. 1646.
    14. Breay, 'Nursing in the Victorian Era', p. 496.
    15. 'The Nursing of the Sick Under Queen Victoria', p. 1646.
    16. Breay, 'Nursing in the Victorian Era', p. 496.
    17. Ibid., p. 496.
    18. 'The Nursing of the Sick Under Queen Victoria', p. 1648.
    19. Breay, 'Nursing in the Victorian Era', p. 493.
    20. Ibid., p. 502.
    21. 'The Nursing of the Sick Under Queen Victoria', pp. 1645–6.
    22. Ibid., p. 1646.
    23. Ibid., p. 1646.
    24. Ibid., p. 1647.
    25. Ibid., p. 1648.
    26. Carr, *What is History?*, p. 12ff.
    27. Ibid., pp. 119–20.
    28. 'Hospital nurses as they are and as they ought to be', *Fraser's Magazine*,
vol. 37 (May 1848), pp. 539–40.
    29. *Medical Times and Gazette*, no. 80, n.s. (10 January 1852), p. 40.
    30. 'The nurse in leading strings', *Household Words* (12 June 1858), pp.
604–5.
    31. Harriet Martineau, 'Women's Battlefield', *Once a Week* (3 December
1859), p. 475.
    32. 'Nurses Wanted', *Cornhill Magazine*, vol. XI (February 1865), pp.
412–14.
    33. John F. South, *Facts Relating to Hospital Nurses* (London, 1857).
    34. Ibid., p. 5.
    35. Ibid., pp. 16–17.
    36. *Guy's Hospital Reports* (edited by Fagge and Durham), vol. XVI, 3rd
series (1871), pp. 541–55. The authorship of the report 'The Nursing Arrangements in Guy's Hospital' in this volume has been attributed to Dr Steele in
'Report of the Nursing Arrangements of the London Hospitals', *British Medical
Journal* (28 February 1874), p. 285.
    37. 'On Nursing Systems', *British Medical Journal*, vol. 1 (3 January 1880),
p. 11.
    38. South, *Facts Relating to Hospital Nurses*, pp. 9–13.
    39. *Guy's Hospital Reports*, pp. 541–3.
    40. South, *Facts Relating to Hospital Nurses*, p. 11.
    41. *Guy's Hospital Reports*, p. 553.
    42. South, *Facts Relating to Hospital Nurses*, p. 17.
    43. *Guy's Hospital Reports*, p. 543.
    44. Ibid., pp. 540–1.
    45. Ibid., pp. 544–5.
    46. South, *Facts Relating to Hospital Nurses*, pp. 12–13, 15.
    47. *Guy's Hospital Reports*, p. 554.
    48. South, *Facts Relating to Hospital Nurses*, pp. 25–6.
    49. Ibid., p. 23.
    50. *Guy's Hospital Reports*, pp. 553–4.
    51. South, *Facts Relating to Hospital Nurses*, p. 28.
    52. This conclusion does not exclude the Institute of Nursing Sisters, nor the

activities of Mrs Fry, from further research into their relation to nursing.

53. St John's House Sisterhood, 'Statement of the Lady Superior addressed to The Right Honourable, the Lord Hatherley'. Privileged communication for Governors of King's College Hospital only (1874), pp. 3–4.

54. *Guy's Hospital Reports*, p. 553.

55. 'Statement of the Lady Superior', p. 5.

56. Ibid., p. 9.

57. Ibid., p. 8.

58. Ibid., p. 8.

59. St John's House – King's College Hospital, 'Hints for Nurses' (n.d.), p. 1.

60. Henry Bonham-Carter, 'Suggestions for Improving the Management of the Nursing Department of Large Hospitals' (1867). It is of importance to note that the training of nurses is not within a training school but within a nursing department of a hospital.

61. Ibid., p. 3.

62. Ibid., p. 8.

63. Ibid., pp. 18–19.

64. Ibid., p. 4.

65. Ibid., p. 9.

66. Ibid., pp. 4–5.

4 THE ADMINISTRATION OF POVERTY AND THE DEVELOPMENT OF NURSING PRACTICE IN NINETEENTH-CENTURY ENGLAND[1]

Mitchell Dean and Gail Bolton

The story of nineteenth-century nursing reform is often told as Florence Nightingale's story of her nurses in the Crimean War, her training schools, her battles for the reform of workhouse nursing and her support of district nursing schemes. Katherine Williams has already shown in the previous chapter the different weight which different writers can put upon these 'facts'. Mitchell Dean and Gail Bolton step further away from a history of individual pioneers. Contemporary political and economic struggles and the contemporary vocabulary for understanding them are the stuff, they argue, of which nursing reform was made. Ideas about sickness were closely intertwined with ideas about poverty, riot and crime and we must make a special effort to understand this unfamiliar mode of conceptualising the world before we can grasp the action which flowed from it. Once we do this, we can understand much better the contradictory position in which nurses historically have found themselves.

Some historians may want to dispute the details of Dean and Bolton's analysis; for there is going on at the moment a reassessment amongst historians as to the character of nineteenth-century social policy and an important debate around the theme of social control. Yet this should not detract attention from the over-all message of this chapter. Can nursing today hope to sustain aims and practices which flow against the tide – and is the modern emphasis on 'caring' facing just this problem? This it seems to me, is the question Dean and Bolton pose for us today.

—————Ed.

The aim of this chapter is to situate the birth of modern nursing practice in the mid-nineteenth century in two ways: first, by drawing on the central themes of the discourses about poverty and the means of its practical administration and, secondly, by tracing various paths by which nursing practice emerged as a technique for the management of the sick poor. In short, nursing practice will be viewed in terms of the social problem of poverty for nineteenth-century reform and policy.

To begin, we discuss the frameworks in which poverty was conceptualised in the early nineteenth century. In these frameworks (political economy and social administration), the field of knowledge produced to deal with poverty reveals the conditions of the emergence of specific domains, targets and means of intervention. In this discussion we seek to elucidate the mode in which the regulation of the population and the management of the poor became of vital political concern in the period in which nursing achieved its modern form.

This general argument, contained in the first section of this chapter, will act as a guide for the analysis of the development of nursing as a means of 'managing' the sick poor and ameliorating the 'danger' to both health and social order inherent in their behaviour and conditions. We take account of the different settings in which care for the sick poor was given – namely, the workhouse, the hospitals, the epidemics and the homes of the poor – so as to show that nursing practice has its historical conditions in the different modes of confinement of the sick poor and in relation to problems of habitation, sanitation and family. To illuminate these historical conditions and to isolate some of the crucial presuppositions of the nursing reformers we have not hesitated to utilise the texts of Florence Nightingale.

The Discourse and Administration of Poverty

In the first part of this chapter, we seek to establish the terms by which poverty was conceptualised in the early nineteenth century. Hence what follows is a discussion of the means of this conceptualisation which is found in the discourses of political economy and social administration. It is our contention that a crucial key to understanding the field of intervention of nursing practice and its object of transformation can only be established by locating it within the broad terrain given in the discussions about poverty which are characteristic of the nineteenth century. In turn, these discussions must be situated within the new forms of political and social organisation which emerge in this period.

Let us start with political economy. There were two elements of this discipline by which we can ascertain the limits of the discourse on poverty throughout the nineteenth century: namely, its discussion of the distribution of wealth in society and of the existence of rich and poor, and the laws by which population growth is regulated.

Political economy, from Adam Smith onwards, sought to enshrine the eternal nature of the rich/poor relationship: 'Wherever there is great property, there is great inequality. For one very rich man, there must be at least 500 poor, and the affluence of the few supposes the indigence of the many.'[2] This statement of Smith, together with the pleas by David Ricardo a half-century later for the abolition of the poor laws, set the register in which this debate was played out.

The question of assistance to the poor was considered by political economy in the following way. The poor rate diverts resources away from capital and thus depresses the production of wealth; hence the more revenue spent on the poor laws, the more the demand for labour will decrease. Furthermore, because at any one time the aggregate wage fund is finite, poor relief will ultimately lower the general level of wages of those employed. Consequently, instead of ameliorating immiseration and poverty, poor relief multiplies the numbers of the poor and increases the sum of misery. Not only that, but the rich, too, shall be so taxed as finally to be transformed into the poor. To quote Ricardo, in evidence of this view:

> The clear and direct tendency of the poor laws . . . is not, as the legislature benevolently intended, to amend the condition of the poor but to deteriorate the condition of both rich and poor; instead of making the poor rich, they are calculated to make the rich poor; and while the present laws are in force, it is quite in the natural order of things that the fund for the maintenance of the poor should progressively increase till it has absorbed all the net revenue of the country.[3]

Coupled with this is the moral view that charity to the poor produces habits in them which are intransigent and which can only be overcome through the enforced acceptance of labour. From this view, labour or the worth of one's own exertions is the great educator of the poor. Ricardo again is informative in this regard:

> The nature of the evil points out the remedy. By gradually contracting the sphere of the poor laws; by impressing on the poor the value of independence, by teaching them that they must look not to systematic or casual charity, but to their own exertions for support, that prudence and forethought are neither unnecessary nor unprofitable virtues, we shall by degrees approach a sounder and more healthful state.[4]

For Ricardo it is the regulation of the labour force by the law of supply and demand which eternises the condition of poverty. For him, it is self-defeating to divert resources away from the rich to the poor. Increasing the wages of the labouring poor above their necessary means of subsistence will create the conditions for an increase in the labouring population. The supply of labourers will increase relative to the demand of capital and, as a result of the increasing competition for jobs, wages will fall and unemployment will result. The natural distribution of wealth, together with the laws of demand and supply, mean the eternal presence of the poor. The poor laws, by making the poor dependent on charity and by teaching the poor imprudence and laziness, legislate against a sound state. They fail to teach the poor the value of labour.

The second crucial concept in the discourses of political economy relevant here is that of 'population'. The concept started to emerge as a central theme at the beginning of the nineteenth century with Thomas Malthus. Its pertinence to our argument is given by its linkage to the question of what should be done about poverty. The crucial aspect to notice is that, while the concept of the 'poor' was not seen as co-terminous with that of the 'population', it was through the conditions of poverty that the growth of population could be regulated. The fundamental principle of Malthus's *Essay on Population* (1798) is pertinent here.

For Malthus, the means of subsistence increase only in arithmetical ratio, while the population, when unchecked, increases in geometrical ratio. But since 'food is necessary for the life of man, the effect of these two unequal powers must be kept equal'.[5] The regulation of these unequal powers is operated by the difficulty of subsistence — that is to say, the scarcity of nature. Therefore, one must not interfere with this natural process by administration of charity. For if we interfere with the conditions of the poor, the population will increase massively. With such a state of population growth, an immiseration of the whole population will occur. The only regulation of the growth of population is, as Malthus said, 'the constant of periodical action of vice and misery'.[6]

Political economy thus posed the problem of the correct means of the government of the poor in a passive fashion: *laissez-faire*. The development of the concept of population was a tool for this dictum which eternalised the condition of the poor and proposed that the best possible intervention was none at all. But what if this mass of the population was to be thrust into such misery that it became a pressing danger to the social order? How was it possible to avert this crisis and not be encouraging the population to grow at an unregulated pace? What had to be resolved was the dictum against interfering with the natural existence of the poor within the population and the desire to promote security, happiness and order.

As a means of formulating these problems, a whole plethora of discourses emerged which linked the question of poverty with the duty of governments to regulate the population. For these discourses which were gradually to delineate the domain proper to the social administration of the poor, the concept of population would furnish a possibility of knowledge of birth and death rates, patterns of dwellings and nutrition, degrees of health and illness. The means of this regulation would, however, be given in terms of techniques and apparatuses applied to individual behaviour and circumstances. It is at this level that, as we shall see, modern forms of nursing practice were to play a vital part. The nurse was to be one element in the rich ensemble of techniques which were elaborated in the later nineteenth century so that the health, sexuality, sanitation and moral behaviour of the population could become an essential part of the art of government. These processes of intervention were not, however, to destroy the distinction of rich and poor, but to preserve it and guarantee the poor's dependence on wage labour as a means of subsistence.

Classical political economy decreed that poverty could not be alleviated. The writings on social administration would decree that the order of state and its wealth could be augmented with practices which attacked not poverty but the dangers contingent upon it and so encouraged a sound population with regulated growth and promoted the highest value in the poor, namely labour. In this respect, it is interesting to note the views of the Poor Law Commissioner, Edwin Chadwick, stating the principles of the Poor Law Amendment Act of 1834, a major turning-point in English administration of poverty: 'The Commissioners might have added that poverty . . . is the natural, the primitive, the general and unchangeable state of man; that as labour is the source of wealth, so is poverty of labour. Banish poverty, you banish wealth.'[7]

In this sense, social administrative practices could remain congruent with political economy. It was not poverty which the Act attempted to remove. As Chadwick stated: 'Poverty . . . was not the object of attack, but rather those circumstances in their environment that turn the poor into the indigent.'[8] There is a particular problematic of poverty here, a distinctive conceptual framework by which questions are posed and answers are produced. This problematic redirects its attention from poverty to its outward manifestations, from the distribution of wealth to moral well-being, from political unrest to the means of order. It is a problematic of the amelioration of detrimental circumstance and dangerous behaviour, not of the existence of poverty. Robert Owen, far from breaking with this conception, is one of its earliest and most forceful exponents:

> In order to effect any radically beneficial change in their character, they the poor must be removed from the influence of such circumstances and placed under those which, being congenial to the natural constitution of man, and the well-being of society, cannot fail to produce that amelioration in their condition, which all classes have so great an interest in promoting.[9]

The conditions of poverty, it was perceived, produced both a moral and political 'danger' to society and social order. Vice and misery, it was conceived, could transform the population into the 'mob'.[10] Owen comments:

> The employer regards the employed as mere instruments of gain while they acquire a gross ferocity of character which if legislative measures should not be devised to prevent its increase, and ameliorate the condition of this class, will sooner or later plunge the country into a formidable and perhaps inextricable state of danger.[11]

An unregulated society thus produces conditions which turn the poor into a danger to society. Government must take an active role in regard to the 'moral improvement' of the poor. For Robert Southey, the influential man of letters and philanthropist, 'There can be no health, no soundness in the state, till government regard the moral improvement of the people as its first duty.'[12]

But what is here called moral improvement must be put into practice at the locality of individual behaviour and character based on what was then a new view of man. Robert Owen, for example, states:

> For instead of the knowledge that the character of man is formed for and not by him being 'one idea' — it will be found to be like the little grain of mustard seed, competent to fill the mind with new and true ideas, and to overwhelm in its consequences all other ideas opposed.[13]

In these discourses we see a whole elaborated system of instruments for the growth and development of this little grain of mustard seed. Southey's detailed proposals are as interesting as his paternalist view of government: improving the local parochial system, a national education system, reform of the police, the development of a savings bank[14] and, importantly for our purposes, the development of Protestant Sisters of Mercy, i.e. a clear voice in favour of a reorganisation of nursing along the lines of the Catholic nuns.[15] But more tellingly than this network of proposals closely detailing the programmes of the mid- and late nineteenth century is the view of how the duty of moral improvement is to be effected by governments.

> Some voluntary castaway there will always be, who no fostering kindness and no parental care preserve from self-destruction, but if any are lost for want of care and culture, there is a sin of omission in the society to which they belong.[16]

Let us examine the nineteenth-century notion of 'care': just as care must be taken for your inanimate machine, so must you care for your living one. Owen's New Lanark project included availability of close medical attention and a system of medical insurance. In these discourses and practices, care is the means by which the conditions likely to produce danger are constantly monitored and kept under control. It is the mode in which the threat to the products of culture is continually suppressed. The business of the nurse, for example, will be that of 'caring' for the sick, preventing all conditions detrimental to the health of the individual and the family, thereby offering a guarantee of the well-being of the population. This process was part of what was termed 'management of the poor'.

Thus, in the mid-nineteenth-century discussions about poverty, a legitimate field of reform and government intervention was worked out. Consider, for example, the problem as it is presented in the 1865 Public Health Report:

> Although my official point of view is one exclusively physical, common humanity requires that the other aspect of this evil should not be ignored . . . In its higher degrees it [overcrowding] almost necessarily involves such negation of all delicacy, such unclean confusion of bodies and bodily functions, such exposure of animal and sexual nakedness, as it is rather bestial than human. To be subject to these influences is a degradation which must become deeper and deeper for those on whom it continues to work. To children who are born under its curse, it must often be a very baptism into infamy. And beyond all measures hopeless is the wish that persons thus circumstanced should ever, in other respects, aspire to that atmosphere of civilisation which has its essence in physical

and moral cleanliness.[17]

In the literature of administration and reform, the image of
'pauperism' provides a referent for all that which necessitates transformation. The above quotation is informed by such an image. In the
'pauper' we find not only the statutory definition of a person who is
forced to accept relief but also a wider connotation as that which is
other to polite, civilised society. Pauperism, in these discourses, stems
from the disorder of bodies and the confusion, both physical and moral,
of bodily functions. As such, pauperism intensifies the communication
of disease and is the breeding ground of delinquency. Its chaos is
opposed to the order of civilisation; its promiscuity is opposed to the
delicacy of polite conduct; its confusion of bodies is opposed to the
correct means of their arrangement and moral behaviour. Indeed, it is so
other than human nature that it belongs, in the order of things, to the
lowest instinctual world of beasts and, as such, the small phrase, the
'management of the poor', carries a specific set of concrete dictates.[18]
If the combating of pauperism formed a general strategic objective in
the nineteenth century, the location of specific tactics of deployment
against it were many. In the next section, the position for the new
nursing practice will be discussed at the sites at which it was invested
with the power of ameliorating pauperism by caring for the sick poor.

The Development of Nursing Practice

Below, we discuss the locations in which nursing practice would be
utilised to effect the transformation of pauperism − namely, the
institutions in which the sick poor were located and also the homes of
the poor. We discuss how nursing reform was situated in the context of
the movement from the confinement of the sick poor in the workhouse
to a general system of hospital care and how the work of the nurse in
the epidemic provides us with a model to comprehend the later
principles.

Workhouse and Hospital

The seventeenth and eighteenth centuries saw the establishment
throughout the twelve to fifteen thousand parishes of institutions for
the paupers. Their purposes were variously designated as industry
houses for the able-bodied, asylums for the infirm and aged, and houses
of correction for vagrants and vagabonds. In practice, however, due to

the economy of the poor rate and the fragmented and tiny character of
parochial administration, any originally intended distinction was rarely
preserved. As the Webbs show, this system 'was always crumbling back
into what the twentieth century terms the General Mixed Workhouse in
which all destitute persons, irrespective of age, sex and condition, all
indiscriminately housed and maintained'.[19]

The tensions inherent in this situation were, if anything, exacerbated
by the Poor Law Amendment Act of 1834. Although it was never
successfully put into practice, all able-bodied applicants were, in
principle, to be refused outdoor relief. The central form of poor relief
available was inside the workhouse and predicated upon the 'less
eligibility' principle. This meant, according to the Poor Law
Commissioners, that the pauper in the workhouse must be in conditions
less favourable than the poorest labourer outside. While the sick and
aged were not meant to be covered by the Act and it was stated in
passing that accommodation might be provided away from the punitive
workhouse buildings, nevertheless the guardians did whatever they
considered most efficient in terms of minimal expenditure of the poor
rate. No clear distinction was made between the able-bodied and the
sick. Abel-Smith remarks that the medical officers did not have the
diagnostic techniques for such a distinction but it should also be noted
that the very structure of the institutional setting militated against it.
The infirmary was hence a part of the workhouse and the 'nurses' there
were called from the ranks of the able-bodied. The workhouse medical
officers held part-time posts, supplementary to their clinical duties in
the early days of private practice, most entering to gain experience in
the lucrative field of midwifery.[20]

On the pauper nurses it is interesting to quote *The Lancet* Sanitary
Commission of 1865, one of the major documents exemplifying the
growing demands for workhouse reforms:

> To make matters as bad as possible, the nurses, with one exception
> are pauper nurses, having improved rations and different dress but
> no pecuniary encouragements. They are mostly a very inferior set of
> women . . . the general character of the nursing will be appreciated
> by the details of the one fact, that we found in one ward two
> paralytic patients with frightful sloughs of the back; they were both
> dirty and lying on hard straw mattresses — the one dressed only with
> a rag steeped in chloride of lime solution, the other with a rag
> thickly covered with ointment. The latter was a fearful and very
> extensive sore, in a state of absolute putridity: the buttocks of the

patient were covered with filth and excoriated and the stench was masked by strewing dry chloride of lime on the floor under the bed. A spectacle more saddening and more discreditable cannot be imagined. Both these patients have since died; no inquest has been held on either.[21]

In articles, reports and commissioners' investigations these 'pauper nurses' are spoken of in singularly disparaging terms: the inferiority of their characters, their agedness, their uncleanliness, their intoxication, their illiteracy and their promiscuity are all that the documentation will allow us to acknowledge of them. Abel-Smith quotes the medical officer of the Strand Workhouse writing in 1859 that 'Such nursing as we had was performed by more or less infirm paupers' and he continues with similar complaints from the head nurse of the Strand Union:

> Of eighteen pauper nurses fourteen were over 60 and four were over 70. Only eight of the eighteen could be relied upon to read the labels on the medicines. Two of them trembled and coughed all day and their combined strength was insufficient to lift a patient up in bed.[22]

When nurses write their own history this period is described as the 'dark ages' of nursing and it is sometimes denied that the pauper nurses had any relation at all to modern nursing practice. But still, nurses they were called, and it was their position which provides a key to the nursing reform movement. The content of criticism of them was to condition the character of the reform that took place.

The shape for interventions, however, was formulated by discussion of nursing reform founded upon the hospital and the generalisation of the hospital system to cater for all the sick poor. This is not to say that the hospital chronologically succeeds the workhouse as the site of confinement of the sick poor. Rather, what we see developing in regard to this particular form of confinement are two parallel sets of institutions and practices represented in the hospital and the workhouse, and the gradual decline of the latter and the expansion of the former. Abel-Smith's account of the hospital system contemporary with the workhouse infirmary is extremely pertinent in this regard.

The situation at the beginning of the century was such that there were five royal hospitals and 57 so-called 'voluntary' hospitals. These hospitals were primarily founded on the beneficence of the rich subscriber to any of the sick poor deemed worthy of entry. In fact, in a

great number of hospitals the subscriber attained the right to nominate
a specific number of entrants and wrote letters of introduction, sat on
the Board of Governors, and was guaranteed contracts for the provision
of its supplies. For the most part, the doctors were selected from the
subscribers' own practitioners and their duties were neither arduous nor
remunerated. In 1820, it was typical for the medical staff to attend
only twice a week. The bulk of the work fell to the resident
'apothecaries' who took charge over the inmates and taught the
apprentices.[23] The matron was, according to Abel-Smith, a subordinate
officer with the charge of the nurses as her main duty. He states that
these early nurses required her close supervision for they were 'little
more than domestic servants of a rather rough and coarse type'.[24]

The hospital as an institution was, however, in the throes of an
important change. Abel-Smith's data reveal that, at least until the
1860s, the voluntary hospital only catered for a minority of the sick.
This work also adduces two key changes during this time. Firstly, the
hospital became a privileged location for the growth and reorganisation
of medical knowledge. It is here that both the widespread dissection of
corpses and a medical knowledge centred on the observation of the
patient were developing. It is here that the modern relation of
observation, research and teaching was being established. It is in the
hospital that specialisation as we know it was forged. Secondly, the
hospital provided the basis for the growth of the realm of intervention
for the medical apparatus. The voluntary hospitals constitute the site
from which medicine was constituted with a new power and nursing
was later to take its modern form.[25]

In a sense, the two sites represent two distinct 'economies'. The
workhouse is a place for the least expensive confinement of those of
the population who add nothing to society's wealth. The labour
performed here is disciplining in that it teaches the idle the value of
their own exertion and useful in so far as it produces something in
return for charity. The hospital, on the other hand, has a somewhat
different economy. Here, medical knowledge and practice form the
investment which the rich constitute for future improvement in the
science of curing. The patients permitted entry were only those of
the poor who were deemed useful for the research and education of the
medical practitioners.[26] In this system of exchanges, the sick poor
offered their bodies for treatment in return not largely for the
possibility of cure but, more simply, for food and habitation. In
return for this they were deprived of their 'freedom' and provided the
raw materials for the accumulation of a special capital, in the shape of

cures for disease. Against this, the cost of their accommodation was small.[27]

The transition from the workhouse infirmary to the hospital as the principal means of curing for the sick poor is a central context in which the movement for nursing reform must be situated. In the workhouse, efficient economy dictated that nursing be assigned to able-bodied paupers; no extra financial outlay was required. In the hospitals, as we shall see below, the nurse is the agency by which constant surveillance, isolation and ordering of patients are carried out. She is the agent by which the conditions which constitute the danger to the health of the population are ameliorated; she is vigilant against an environment conducive to infection and constantly engaged in maintaining that harmony of bodies which alone produces recovery. The economy of the workhouse had dictated its place as a breeding ground of moral and physical danger. The 'curative economy' of the hospital placed discipline, regulation, normalisation and observation first, thereby creating a moral universe in which the sick poor were to lead their existence. The nurse was to be crucial to this new hospital order, as we discuss further below.

The Hospital Order

The status of the new hospital nurse in the hierarchy dominated by the physician is low but, as a transmitter of this most valuable power, she must be distinguished from the sick poor from whom she cares. Not only does she economise on the time of the doctor, but her position is a resolution of the economy of disciplinary power.

In the hospital the nurse must be:

1. in every way, distinguished from that which her practice is designed to transform (viz. the sickness, disharmony and chaos of pauperism);
2. a transmitter of a power which corrects the behaviour attendant upon pauperism, in order to provide moral order;
3. a subordinate within the medical apparatus to sister, matron and doctor.

In the first sense, there is occasioned not only a hierarchy between nurse and patient, but a measure by which the new nursing practice can be distinguished from the 'pauper nursing' and the older type of 'domestic servant' hospital nurses. This was to be effected by a rigorous class-based selection process. In the second, her appearance and behaviour were such that she was the converse of the danger her position sought to ameliorate. This was to be effected through her background, her training and strict discipline. In the third, she must be 'obedient' and 'trustworthy'. The means by which this was to be effected were her training, the definition of her occupation, and continuous supervision.

In the (1881) memorandum for the qualification and admission to the Nightingale Fund Training School we find that: 'The ordinary probationers are intelligent well-educated young women of upper servant class, daughters of small farmers, tradesmen, artisans, etc.'[28]

The class criterion guaranteed that the prospective nurses would not come from the same ranks as the 'rough domestic servants' or the paupers, upon whom the nursing in the workhouse had been based.[29] The new nurse would ideally come from a family of moderate means with a sound education. She would have learnt the value of exertion from her family background but not be without some indirect experience of pauperism. Her lower-middle-class location could be reproduced in the hospital hierarchy.

The class criterion only provided the raw material in order to distinguish the new nursing practice. The other means were the ones of outward significance and morally correct training. If nursing were to play its role in the management of the poor and the eradication of pauperism, it required that these respectable women be subjected to a regime of discipline in their training. The same order that would be lived in the nurses' lives would be imposed on the life of the infirm, on the body of the patients, on the organisation of the ward and the homes of the poor. Florence Nightingale stated:

> Writers on sick nursing have repudiated training without saying what training is . . . we require that a woman be sober, honest, truthful, without which there is no foundation to build. We train them in the habits of punctuality, quietness, trustworthiness, personal neatness. We teach her how to manage the concerns of a large ward or establishment . . . We teach her how to manage helpless patients . . . the management of convalescents: and how to observe the sick and maimed patients.[30]

The nurse's sense of order was ensured by the discipline which was imposed upon her appearance. The uniform was a signifier of her power. Its starched whiteness corresponded to the tasks by which health is maintained and disease prevented. The timepiece was a symbol of the finitude of life and the necessity of using every moment to provide the conditions for its extension. The lack of adornments showed the altruistic zeal of her 'good works'. She would not only care for the bodies of the sick, but through her own body she would become a symbol of the true spiritual requirements of health and the means by which moral rectitude and correct behaviour eradicate the pauperism of disease.

Florence Nightingale's writings are also an enduring indication of the position of the nurse in the transformed hospital system. Against the confusion of pauperism within the workhouse, the hospital, for Nightingale, had to be based on strict order or what Rosenberg has recently called a 'moral universe'.[31] In other words, a series of techniques were to be utilised in order to ensure correct moral behaviour. The principles by which order was introduced were these:

1. the bodies of the patients must be so arranged as to facilitate the surveillance of nurses;
2. observation must be conducted on a strict hierarchical system, for even the nurses must be under the constant supervision of their superiors;
3. the architectural requirements were to be those in which the smallest number of nurses could attend the greatest number of patients.

Nightingale incorporated these rationales in her famous *Notes on Hospitals*: 'There are four essential points of construction as regards nursing and discipline. First; *Economy as to Attendance* . . . secondly, *Ease of Supervision* . . . third and fourth, *Distribution of Sick in convenient numbers for Attendance and Position of Nurses' Rooms* . . .'[32]

The new hospital must be an architectural form which manifests the principles of sanitation and defeats those 'hospital diseases' so common in the infirmaries. In the hospital, the removal of physical barriers in order was a prerequisite to moral intervention. It is here that we can agree with Rosenberg's characterisation of the hospital as 'moral universe'. The central axis around which this moral universe was arranged was the body of the patient. Rosenberg states this well:

The body was visualised in terms of a central metaphor, one in which the organism was seen as a dynamic system constantly interacting with its environment. Diet, atmosphere and ventilation, psychic stress, all interacted to shape a patterned but continuously re-established reality. Within this framework of explanation, disease was no specific entity . . . but rather a general state of disequilibrium.[33]

It is an interesting historical paradox that at the time when medicine was 'discovering' disease in local lesions in the three-dimensional body, nursing and public health were basing themselves on this entirely different model. Moreover, as the opinion of medicine was dissociating the causation of disease from social conditions, nursing and hospital reform was carried out on a theory which made disease peculiarly social. What we are witnessing is two discourses which in isolation are internally coherent and which enable different interventions to be interwoven in the complementary practices of 'cure and treatment' and 'care and prevention'. These two types of knowledge permitted an intervention on the body of the patient which was not only on its physical existence or on its social conditions but upon both at the same time. The medical ensemble in the hospital could intervene at the intersection of the social and the biological, on behaviour as well as on organs and tissue.

Above all, the position of the nurse in the hospital was to be, in the terms of the arguments of Nightingale and the reformers, in every way different from the position of the able-bodied pauper nurse in the workhouse. This must help to explain the great alliances between the hospital and nursing reformers of the 1860s and the concern of nursing reformers with the detail of hospital planning, construction and administration. The changes between the new nursing practice and the pauper nurses are inscribed in the materiality of this dramatic institutional transformation. It was the same points of attack in each case and it was the same principles by which hospital and nursing reform sought to achieve their aims.

The Epidemic and Home Nursing

If, however, we are to limit the context of nursing practice to its place in the new general system of institutional confinement represented by the hospital, some of its features remain unintelligible. For a more complete understanding of the theoretical relation between correct behaviours and the prevention of disease, we must look at the fashion in which the epidemic figures in the medicalisation of poverty. In turn we must recognise that the position of the nurse in the epidemics prefigures her function as a visitor in the homes of the poor. What is central in the discourse on epidemics and the action taken against them brings us back to the major thread of our argument, i.e. the awareness that medical intervention could be a significant form of combating pauperism by policing the poor in the management of their conditions and behaviour.

The major group interested in public health in the period 1830–1860 consisted of the Benthamite 'sanitarians' of Drs Arnott and Kay and especially Southwood Smith, together with the administrator, Edwin Chadwick. Amongst this group, particular stress was given to a multi-causal environmental model of the aetiology of epidemics which the sanitarians viewed as intimately connected with the insanitary conditions of the urban poor. In fact, the term 'sanitary' was still a novelty when utilised in the titles of the reports of Arnott, Kay and Southwood Smith in 1838 and by Edwin Chadwick in 1842. They had linked disease and crime and spoke of the existence of 'fever nests' and 'ghettos' where the outbreaks of epidemic and crime were likely to occur.[34]

The way in which the aetiology of epidemics was conceived by the most publicly successful group in British medicine required a specific political role for medical intervention. Public health, in their conception, must be organised in such a way that a general form of surveillance, recording and control of the 'labouring population' could be practised at the level of individual behaviour and administered on a national scale. We shall illustrate this point below with respect to the position of nurses in the cholera epidemics, which was to serve as a model for future practice.

The sanitarians advocated sanitary improvement as a panacea for physical and social ills. It is difficult to read Chadwick's report or the Health of Towns Association speeches[35] without being struck by their improving zeal. At one meeting of the association, a memorial to a poor doctor who died of fever is recorded. According to Chadwick he died, like many others, in the course of providing maps of the 'habitat of typhus' which demonstrated the 'coincidence with the track of cholera and other epidemics'. Moreover, these maps, he claimed, show conclusively the correspondence of epidemics 'with bad drainage, filth, over-crowding and bad ventilation'.[36] In his speech on the same occasion, Southwood Smith chastised the London Corporation for opposing the introduction of a sanitary bill in Parliament in these terms: '. . . if they pictured in their imagination the suffering that must precede death, and the destitution and pauperism that must follow it, would they entertain any thoughts of obstructing a government anxious to terminate this national calamity'.[37]

These speeches, like the 1842 report, display a similar concern for the relation between epidemics and pauperism or what Chadwick saw as coincidence of pestilence and moral disorder. It is not poverty which multiplies the spread of the epidemic, but the physical conditions of the poor which are conducive to their unclean behaviours. Without physical improvements in sanitation, housing and ventilation, moral agencies were seen to have only a remote chance of success. The advocacy of 'sanitary' improvement was on the dual grounds of facilitating the availability and quality of the labour force and promoting what Chadwick calls 'moral and political conditions'. The 1842 report sums it up well:

> The facts indicated will suffice to show the importance of moral and political considerations viz. that the noxious physical agencies depress the health and bodily condition of the population, and act as obstacles to education and to moral culture; that in abridging the duration of the adult life of the working classes, they check the growth of productive skill and abridge the amount of social experience and steady moral habits in the community; that they substitute for a population that accumulates and preserves instruction and is steadily progressive, a population that is young, inexperienced, ignorant, credulous, irritable, passionate and dangerous.[38]

Nightingale, far from being opposed to the political forces for public health, was firmly on the side of the sanitarians. Charles Rosenberg sees her rejection of contagion theory as a result of the morally resonant polarities of Nightingale's mind.[39] Be that as it may, it seems apparent that this 'mind' was formed in a far wider social and discursive network and that Nightingale's own work is deeply embedded in the materiality of the public health reform movement and is a necessary consequence of the mode of conceptualisation of the realm of intervention in the nineteenth century. She relies heavily on the assumption of the correlation between population density and sickness and she cites four conditions which contribute to disease (all completely consistent with sanitarianism). They are: agglomeration of sick under one roof, deficiency of space per bed, deficiency of fresh air, deficiency of light. Nor is it surprising that she should term preventive domestic nursing as 'sanitary nursing'.[40]

For nursing, the work in the epidemic is the model of an intervention to be conducted at the level of the individual and family. The use of nurses to this end was not of universal moment but the success with which they were used in the 1850s indicates the terms in which the nurse's relation to the domestic situation place her as a valuable part of the management of the population in later times. Where the nurse was called on to intervene, e.g. the 1854 cholera epidemic, her 'care' was revealed as a crucial link in the fight against the 'danger' represented by the physical conditions of the poor in their own homes.

This role is clearly exemplified in Sir William Acland's memoirs of the 1854 cholera outbreak in Oxford.[41] In this epidemic, nurses were engaged to carry out the local Board of Guardians' decision that medical attendance should be provided at the houses of the poor. Their selection was made on the advice of the local churchmen to the Oxford Board of Guardians. The Acland memoirs retell:

> In the Police Office . . . a list was kept of all the respectable women who were willing to nurse in Cholera houses. The names had been furnished mainly through the local knowledge of their parochial clergy . . . After they had nursed three nights they were allowed a day's rest and the option of going again to nurse . . . When a new Case of Cholera was announced in the house of any poor person, a Messenger from the Police Office proceeded to the house of a Nurse 'returned home', and sent her to the place at which her help was required. It was then the business of an Inspector . . . to go there, to ascertain whether the interior economy of the house was such that the order of the Medical Attendant could be followed. If not, his duty was to forward from the Police Office the deficiency: food, bedding, blankets, hot bottles &c. And lastly, because the most important, a lady visited every house to instruct the nurses to comfort the sick, to cheer the disconsolate and, where need was, herself to supply a sudden emergency, or to relieve a wearied attendant.[42]

The epidemic was used by Acland to argue for the necessity of providing nurses to attend the poor in their own homes. He argued that this body of competent women could, at all times, wait on the poor who had been pauperised by infirmity. This is a suggestion that has indeed come quite a long way since 1854! Not only would these women be necessary in times of epidemic, but they could be on guard against the conditions of pauperism which are known to be favourable to the origin and intensification of disease. For this reason it was said that these nurses would be of great benefit not only for the poor but for all classes in society.

In the accounts of the epidemics, we see for the first time the administrative use of nurses as an over-all technique of intervention based on visits to the homes of the poor. We find that nursing in an epidemic required the 'moral qualities' that became so crucial to the cause of nursing reform. So much was this so that one account recalls the popular saying 'it takes a good woman to be a good nurse'.[43] How far the administrative intervention of nursing for the poor in their homes has come since these humble beginnings is another matter; the point here is that the terms in which this was to happen were, at least partly, shaped by the ubiquitous spectre of the epidemic.

In the writings of the mid-nineteenth-century reformers, the presence of the epidemic and the workhouse linked disease to its social conditions. Disease, the otherness inside the human body, was linked to 'pauperism', the otherness inside the social body. The central task for nursing was one of preventing the possibilities of physical disease, by watching over the poor and ameliorating the moral disease of pauperism.

Where the Benthamite sanitarians had built sanitation and public health demands upon the image of pauperism and all that this image evoked, the same language can be found in the most famous works of Florence Nightingale. Again, the insanitary dark quarters of the poor, their lack of morality and decency and their ignorance are the elements which are seen as conducive to infection and disease. In *Notes on Nursing* (1859), Nightingale stated that the spread of disease was linked to the density of population, to the vapours which carried infection in the unhygienic darkness of their rooms, to the lack of ventilation, to their noise and confusion, to inadequate diet, to lack of cleanliness of walls and floor, to the unhelpful chattering and advice, to their unhealthy bed and bedding, and so on. But perhaps the most important lesson which the relation between paupers, disease and epidemic conveyed to the nursing reformers in general, and to Nightingale in particular, was the need for meticulous observation as a means of prevention and care. This 'need' was to be fulfilled within their vision of a reformed nursing practice.

The lesson they learnt was that in order to break the chaos of disease in the human body careful observation must be taken of its social conditions. In the epidemics the most progressive medical boards hired nurses to watch over the sick and thereby to ensure that the behaviour of the sick was neither detrimental to recovery nor conducive to further infection. It was important to discipline bodies by isolating them in the quarantine of their rooms or to remove them to better conditions, to make sure the premises were clean, hygienic and disinfected, to be ever on watch, as Nightingale said, 'against want of cleanliness, foul air, want of light and warmth'.[44]

The care of the sick by nurses during the epidemics had followed these sanitary doctrines and formed a testing ground for a system of inspection and surveillance. As a central figure in the organised management of the population in times of epidemic, the position of the nurse as a visitor to the homes of the poor and as a means of control and prevention was given a certain validity. Now, while there is little evidence which suggests a direct link between epidemic nursing and the later district nursing, the similarities between the formulation of the tasks of the latter and the model of the former are striking. We shall use Nightingale's writings to demonstrate this connection. Just as nursing in the epidemic combated the disorderly behaviour and conditions favourable to the spread of the disease, so the district nurse could be the agency of an order calculated to watch over the potential chaos emanating from the poor. Where epidemic nursing had sought to prevent the intensification and multiplication of the disease, the district nurse would prevent disease and alleviate its effects at the very origin. To do this, the district nurse must teach the poor the correct manner of living:

> Besides nursing the patient, she shows them in their own home, how they can help in this nursing, how they can be clean and orderly, how they can improve appliances, how their home need not be broken up . . . the district nurse may be the forerunner in teaching the disorderly how to use improved dwellings — teaching without seeming to teach, which is the ideal of teaching.[45]

For the proponents of district nursing, exemplified in Nightingale, the nurse in the community was, with almost missionary zeal, to monitor the constant danger of pauperism; she was to dispel its ignorance by teaching; she was to demonstrate how its filth could be combated; she was to transform disorder and insanitation into order and cleanliness. But above all she could supervise the family in order that the burdens of child-bearing and child-rearing, or of an injured breadwinner, be accepted without breaking up the home.

The district nurse was to become in the latter part of the century an insurance of the state against the moral and physical danger which pauperised the poor and facilitated the dissolution of the family. Against the unclean promiscuity which attached to the image of pauperism, and the consequent threat which the moral disorder of bodies was seen to pose, the regulated sexuality of the family was becoming the means by which political docility was ensured. The family, in its improved dwellings with adequate sanitation, was to be supervised by visitors to the poor.

What has been outlined above are the general features of the way in which nursing reform can be seen to have been located as a system of providing care for the sick poor in relation to the discursive and practical conditions of administration and management, in terms of theories and aims of sanitarianism and in the transformations occurring in medicine and confinement. As such, this chapter should be viewed as opening up a wide field of problems rather than as a recitation of linear events. However, it should be noted that, as Brian Abel-Smith has lucidly shown, the movements for nursing, public health and hospital reform provided specific instances where their alliance was crucial to the development of a new relation between the state and health. The 1850s and 1860s are particularly interesting in this regard. Here we see the great confluence of nursing reformers, like Nightingale and Louisa Twining, poor law doctors, sanitarian-inspired poor law officers and inspectors, as well as influential philanthropic reformers, providing the base for workhouse and poor law reform agitation which led to the 1867 Metropolitan Poor Act. The Act, as Abel-Smith said, provided 'the first explicit acknowledgement that it was the duty of the state to provide hospitals for the poor' and, as such, 'was an important step toward the National Health Service Act which followed some 80 years later'.[46]

Conclusion

The conditions which made modern nursing practice possible were created in a common struggle over the correct means of administration of the sick poor. The system of the new nursing practice and the terms in which reforms were made existed within a common discourse based on the transformation of pauperism by specific principles of sanitation and institutional confinement and a specific view of how the poor ought to behave, whether in their own homes or as patients in the hospital. But why did reform of the medical apparatus and the position of nursing practice within it take this particular form?

We have argued that to understand these features it is necessary to return to the discourses in which nursing reform and practice are delineated and to situate these in the wider context of the formulations of poverty and its means of administration. In this way we can reconstruct the aim, objective and means of nursing practice and situate it in the attempts to forge forms of administrative apparatus, types of intervention and a new specific relation of the poor to the state.

As we have repeatedly stressed throughout this chapter, the discourse on social administration is an attempt to provide a technical apparatus for the control of what it saw as a danger. The emergent state was slowly being constituted as the locus of the amelioration of this danger by a series of interventions upon its conditions. None of the strategies incorporated in the state sought, in any way, to tamper with the causes of poverty and the capitalist division of labour. None of them sought even to conceptualise what the causes of poverty might be! The discourses on poverty are discourses on the best means of its conservation, and not of its alleviation, for poverty is viewed as essential to the production of wealth.

The position of the new nursing practice can be viewed in the context of the development, in the nineteenth century, of a macro-politics of the 'population' along with the micro-politics of bodies and behaviour. It is here that we can locate the relation of nursing practice both to the sick poor, on the one hand, and to the emergent state, on the other. Improved sanitation, hygiene, habitation and health were considered at the level of effects on the whole population. There, the threat to the new social order is averted by measures which affect all the population at once, e.g. the construction of a sanitation system and a central health administration. On the other hand, in the micro-political system, a surveillance, recording and disciplining of the behaviour and bodies occur so that detrimental and chaotic conduct may be modified. The agency of nursing practice is one of the means by which 'danger' is averted at this level and by which 'care' of the individual produces docile subjects in a relation of dependence to the state.[47]

The micro-political system acts as an effective relayer of knowledge through the administrative apparatus. Thus the nurse, for example, helps constitute a politics of the population by her role in the collection of information. She systematically registers, observes, monitors and records her target of intervention, whether in the domestic or hospital scenes. On the other side of this interchange, measures which are undertaken at the level of the population necessitate a large number of techniques for implementation and a vast number of agents to put them into effect. At the point of contact with the individual the nurse is paradoxically ensuring the well-being of the population. It is here, with the family, as with the patient, that the possibility of a moral and health threat to the social order is defused.

Caught within this interchange of population and individual health, population and domestic sanitation, population and familial sexuality and child-rearing, the nurse constantly finds herself in a contradictory position. She is one of the agents of a power which is constantly operating in her own training and activity. As she supervises the patient or the family, she is overseen by her superiors. In the historical constitution of nursing practice every effort was taken to ensure that the nurse would remain the model of a disciplinary, obedient individual. This was necessary if she was to become the last link in a chain of the power which sought the correction and transformation of behaviours and conditions. Her intervention was to constitute that absolutely delicate point by which the administration of the population would meet the locality of bodies, their health and their sexuality.

Certainly, the state's assumption of a duty to care for the sick poor answers the demands of capital for a certain type of labour force. Nevertheless, interwoven with economic 'necessity', this duty is effected in such a way that individuals are placed in a network of power which makes them both dependent on the state and constantly policed by it. This is the major co-ordinate which structures every encounter of nurse and patient, nurse and family.

All the strivings of the nurse are conditioned in this way. As one of the dominated classes, her position is constituted in a network of disciplinary practices. As an agent of the transmission of power, her own daily practice is designed to produce docile subjects and to render harmless the tensions within the family and those exacerbated by sickness. It is, moreover, the contradictory nature of her position that may indicate possibilities for an alternative role.

This chapter is a contribution to the location of nursing in modern society and to the genesis of what we now recognise as nursing practice. We have tried to open up a realm of debate which concentrates on the inscription of nursing in forms of power which characterise our society and its government. The specific nature of nursing as an agency of the correction of behaviours and disciplining of bodies, as a technique of intervention against not only health danger but also moral and social dangers, as an apparatus of the administration of certain sections of the population, as a crucial link between the state and the poor and as a regulator of health, habitation and family life, cannot be disregarded if we are to understand the complexity of relationships through which nursing is assigned a position in modern society. In short, we are hoping to encourage debate on all the functions of nursing which comprise this history. Nursing, even today, cannot be considered as external to the techniques and agencies of the forms of power which constitute our administrative machinery. The nurse, as a key position of transmission of this power, can call its forms into question and open the possibility of a new politics of health and a new domain of struggle.

Notes

1. This chapter is a revised version of a paper delivered by the authors at the BSA Medical Sociology Conference at the University of York in October 1979.

2. A. Smith, *An Enquiry into the Nature and Causes of the Wealth of Nations* (edited by R. N. Campbell and A. S. Skinner), 2 vols (Oxford University Press, London, 1976), p. 710.

3. D. Ricardo, *The Principles of Political Economy and Taxation* (edited by P. Sraffa) (Cambridge University Press, London, 1962), pp. 105–6.

4. Ibid., p. 15.

5. T. Malthus, *An Essay on the Principle of Population as it Effects the Future Improvement of Society*, 1st edn (Johnson, London, 1798), p. 11.

6. Ibid., p. 15.

7. E. Chadwick, *An Article on the Principles and Progress of the Poor Law Amendment Act*, British Museum Tracts (Charles Knight, London, 1837), p. 18.

8. Ibid., p. 42.

9. R. Owen, 'Report to the Committee of the Association of the Manufacturing and Labouring Poor', published in *Tracts on Social Reform* (Longman, Hurst, Rees and Orme, London, 1818), p. 13.

10. G. Pearson, *The Deviant Imagination* (Macmillan, London, 1975); see Ch. 6: 'The Historical Object of Deviance: King Mob'.

11. R. Owen, *Observations on the Effects of the Manufacturing System* (Longman, Hurst, Rees and Orme, London, 1815), p. 5.

12. R. Southey, *Sir Thomas More or the Colloques on the Progress and Prospects of Society*, vol. 2 (London, 1829), p. 424, quoted in R. Williams, *Culture and Society, 1780–1950* (Penguin, Harmondsworth, 1963), p. 42.

13. R. Owen, *The Life of Robert Owen by Himself* (London, 1920), p. 105, quoted in Williams, *Culture and Society*, p. 46.

14. Ibid., p. 43.

15. Southey, *Sir Thomas More*, p. 318.

16. Ibid., p. 425.

17. Quoted by K. Marx, *Capital: A Critique of Political Economy*, vol. 1 (translated by E. Aveling and S. Moore) (Charles Kerr and Co., Chicago, 1915), p. 723.

18. We are well aware that the development of techniques and discourse dealing with the management of pauperism and the administration of the poor in the period 1790–1860 is intimately connected with the shift of the balance of class forces and the ascendant hegemony of the industrial capitalist class. The real threat posed by the popular classes in the city and countryside has been extensively covered by E. Hobsbawm, *Industy and Empire* (Penguin, Harmondsworth, 1969) (especially pp. 64–8) and the revolutionary potential posed by working-class organisation is detailed in E. P. Thompson, *The Making of the*

English Working Class (Penguin, Harmondsworth, 1963) (see p. 194ff). It seems that this threat was exacerbated even further by the inability of the landowning governing class to provide effective political direction, and the strict dichotomy between repression (e.g. Anti-Combination Acts, 'Peterloo', etc.) and benevolence (e.g. the Speenhamland relief system of the 1790s). To extrapolate from our argument it may be said that the industrial capitalist hegemony based itself, at least partially, on a practice of administration which linked practical control to assistance and welfare in order to place the masses of the people in a dominated but orderly position in the new system. Indeed, the concern with poverty in this period is the key to the dramatic reorganisation of the whole government machinery which is witnessed in the nineteenth century; see also H. Perkin, *The Origins of Modern English Society 1780–1900* (Routledge and Kegan Paul, London, 1969).

19. S. and B. Webb, *English Poor Law History: Part One, The Old Poor Law* (Longmans, Green and Co., London, 1927), p. 218.

20. B. Abel-Smith, *The Hospitals 1800–1948: A Study in Social Administration in England and Wales* (Heinemann, London, 1964), Ch. 4, especially pp. 45–57.

21. '*The Lancet* Sanitary Commission for Investigation into the State of the Infirmaries of Workhouses', *The Lancet*, 12 August 1865, p. 188.

22. B. Abel-Smith, *A History of the Nursing Profession* (Heinemann, London, 1960), p. 11.

23. Abel-Smith, *The Hospitals*, pp. 4–8 and 46ff.

24. Ibid., p. 8.

25. Ibid., pp. 4, 21–3 (specialisation), pp. 16–18 (on research and teaching), Ch. 5.

26. Ibid., pp. 12–15, 46.

27. For a parallel type of account of similar processes in France see M. Foucault, *The Birth of the Clinic: An Archaeology of Medical Perception* (translated by A. M. Sheridan) (Tavistock, London, 1976), Ch. 5.

28. Quoted by A. Austin, *History of Nursing Source Book* (G. P. Putnam's Sons, New York, 1957), p. 270.

29. Pauper nursing was put to a formal end in August 1897 by the Local Government Board after some 50 years of the movement of nursing reform. For further discussion see G. Bolton and M. Dean, 'Questioning Nursing History', in *Nursing Mirror* (forthcoming).

30. F. Nightingale, 'Una and the Lions', in *Good Words* (London, 1 June 1868), p. 360, reprinted in Austin, *Source Book*.

31. C. Rosenberg, 'Florence Nightingale on Contagion: The Hospital as a Moral Universe', in C. Rosenberg (ed.), *Healing and History* (Dawson, New York, 1979).

32. F. Nightingale, *Notes on Hospitals*, 3rd edn (Longmans, London, 1863), pp. 50–1.

33. Rosenberg, 'Florence Nightingale on Contagion', p. 117.

34. M. Pelling, *Cholera, Fever and English Medicine 1825–1865* (Oxford University Press, Oxford, 1978), Chs 1 and 2. Pelling admirably demonstrates that this position was in stark contrast to the increasingly local mono-causal contagion theories of French origin which were increasingly influential in England.

35. E. Chadwick, *Report on an Inquiry into the Sanitary Conditions of the Labouring Population* (HMSO, 1842), and E. Chadwick *et al.*, *Health of Towns* (Chapman, Elcoate and Co., London, 1847).

36. Chadwick *et al.*, *Health of Towns*, p. 4.

37. Ibid., p. 14.

38. Chadwick, *Report*, p. 132.

39. Rosenberg, 'Florence Nightingale on Contagion', p. 124.

40. Nightingale, *Notes on Hospitals*; F. Nightingale, *Notes on Nursing* (Harrison, London, 1859).

41. Sir H. W. Acland, *Memoir of the Cholera Epidemic at Oxford in 1854* (Churchill, London, 1856), pp. 98–9.

42. Ibid., p. 101.

43. E. C. Richards, *Felicia Skene of Oxford: A Memoir* (Murray, London, 1902), p. 111; see also M. Goodman, *Experiences of a Sister of Mercy* (South Elder, London, 1862).

44. Nightingale, *Notes on Nursing*, p. 71.

45. From the Introduction to W. Rathbone's *Sketch of the History and Progress of District Nursing* (London, 1890), quoted in Austin, *Source Book*.

46. Abel-Smith, *The Hospitals*, p. 82. For his extremely lucid account of the agitation which led to the 1867 Act, see Ch. 5.

47. It should be mentioned that the recent work of Michel Foucault provided the impetus for many of the themes of this chapter. No explicit references have been made to these texts simply because it would be impossible to account for what this chapter owes to them. None the less, his work should be brought to the attention of those nursing historians who wish to elaborate on any of the problems raised in this chapter; cf. *History of Sexuality Volume One: An Introduction* (translated by R. Hurley) (Allen Lane, London, 1979), and *Discipline and Punish: The Birth of the Prison* (translated by A. Sheridan) (Allen Lane, London, 1977).

5 A CONSTANT CASUALTY: NURSE EDUCATION IN BRITAIN AND THE USA TO 1939

Celia Davies

Nursing history textbooks are strangely global; they shift with apparent
ease from Kaiserswerth in Germany to the London of Miss Nightingale
and then, because they are mostly American textbooks, to developments in the USA. In one way this is justified, for nursing is international
and ideas from one country are quickly taken up in others. In another
way it is less fortunate, for we fail to appreciate the advantages of a
deliberate cross-cultural comparison. I have chosen nurse education in
Britain and the USA as my topic in this chapter for two main reasons.
First, I find that many nurses are critical of provision for nurse
education in Britain, but feel especially powerless to change it. I hope
that this comparative perspective helps explain why. Secondly, I think
these same nurses sometimes look enviously across the Atlantic. Not
only do I think that the business of transplants here as elsewhere is
fraught with difficulty, but I also want to suggest that the American
pattern has its disadvantages too.

There are those who will wish for a more detailed account of
British nursing education and one which comes up to date. Certainly I
find myself in agreement with this sentiment, and frustrated that nurse
education has somehow been the subject-matter but not the real
subject of historical writings. My aim here, however, has not been to
cover a period, but to highlight the utility of cross-cultural comparisons.
I must leave the reader to judge whether this was the right decision
given the present state of our knowledge and understanding.

————Ed.

Education requires resources. Sufficiently powerful people must believe
sufficiently in the worth of allocating resources to education if
anything is to change. It is not just a matter of a budget to pay
teachers; it is a matter also of providing equipment and facilities, of
releasing learners for the classroom, of teaching potential teachers to
teach and, if the learning is of a vocational sort, of interrupting the
daily practice of the skill in order to provide opportunity for learners to
learn. This chapter traces solutions to these problems in the field of
nursing in Britain and the USA. It deals with a period from the late
nineteenth century to the 1940s and it focuses on education for the
status of qualified nurse.[1]

At first sight, American nurses appear more favourably placed.
University and collegiate courses have long been a feature of the
American scene, and a fair proportion of nurses in the US can hope to

ascend a career ladder in the field of nurse education even to the
position of professor. Nurse education, it seems, has been allocated
resources, and the problem is to understand why we in Britain are less
favoured. The position taken here, however, is more complex than this.
I shall argue that both American and British nursing education have
been starved of resources, though in different ways, and that economic
and political interests in each case have intruded to the disadvantage of
nurses. I shall also try to show how these different institutional patterns
have shaped the experience of nurses, the way in which they have
interpreted their worlds and the demands they have made.

What follows, then, is a comparative account of the development of
patterns of nurse education in Britain and the USA. It is a story, in
both settings, of compromise — a compromise involving minimal
resources to education. At the outset similar solutions were found in
both countries; it was thereafter that the differences really began to
surface. British and American nurses organised themselves differently
and fought different battles in different arenas. These differences help .
us to understand why conflicts cooled down in the British case and
heated up in the American. We leave the story at a point where British
nurses could barely envisage change, whereas their counterparts in the
USA, though they could envisage it, could not accomplish it.

The 'Take-off' in Nursing Education

This is not the place to document the many and diverse local efforts in
Britain and America in the nineteenth century to improve nursing and
to implement some form of training for recruits.[2] Certainly Miss
Nightingale was not the first to implement such an idea. Her system
requires scrutiny here, however, for two reasons: first, because she
herself was so influential and charismatic a figure; secondly, because the
system contained within it a means for its transmission to other sites
and settings.

The major features of Florence Nightingale's system of training for
nurses, put into practice at St Thomas' Hospital in 1860 and thereafter
taken elsewhere by its students, are familiar.[3] Recruits to the school
worked in the hospital under the watchful eye and rule-making genius
of the matron. The remit of their duties was wide for they were to do
whatever was necessary for the well-being of patients and the smooth
running of the hospital. Their training was essentially practical and
they learned on the job. Their conduct and character were subject to

scrutiny both in the wards and outside their work. This latter was circumscribed by the rules of the nurses' home and the surveillance of the home sister. The matron did some of the teaching but most of the lectures (in off-duty time) were given by the doctors on the staff of the hospital. The school, unlike many, was independently funded, and probationers contracted their loyalty to the Nightingale Fund. After a single training year they agreed to work wherever the fund should send them for a further three years. It was this which gave Miss Nightingale and her trustees a supply of trained nurses to send, in groups, to implement the Nightingale system.

What is important about this for the present argument is that it represented a minimal allocation of resources and a minimal change in the *status quo*. There was no 'school' in the sense of an independent entity with an attached staff and pupils who saw formal learning as their major life commitment. There was no developed body of specialist knowledge available and ready to be transmitted. There was no general acceptance that teaching and learning roles were so self-evidently legitimate that they should command resources. The Nightingale strategy of nurse education in effect meant the staffing of hospitals with a strictly disciplined labour force of probationers. They would do the work of the hospital both uncomplainingly and cheaply. Miss Nightingale's conception of what the nurse was and should be provided a rationale and justification for this. Furthermore, when a specialised teaching role did come, it came as an adjunct to teaching by the sister in the ward. Nor did the tutor, as she was called, lecture the students: hers was a much lowlier position than that of the medical lecturers. She attended lectures, corrected students' notes on them and reworked material when students encountered difficulty.

This form of nursing education was a compromise based on the existing institutional framework of the hospital. It neither challenged the doctors' status nor made demands on the hospital administrators for resources. It could probably only have worked in a world where women were prepared to be so self-denying, so hard-working and so amenable to discipline. Nineteenth-century England, with its lack of job opportunities for women, was such a world.[4] Even so, doctors and those responsible for the running of the hospitals were suspicious. A great deal of persuasion was necessary to allow experiments to get under way at all; and doctors in particular were watchful for anything which challenged their interests. But the Nightingale compromise did catch on, not just in the sense of the growing army of Nightingales across the globe,[5] but in the much more important sense, for our purposes, of

probationer staffing. A system of nurse education conceived in this
fashion made political and economic sense in the hospitals. Strictly
controlled as they were by the matron, the nurses were disciplined
workers; and the matron's anxiety to prove the value of nurses meant
that firm discipline was vital to her. While providing living quarters for
probationers was an outlay for the hospital, it was repaid in the
smaller stipend payable and the availability and accessibility of the
workforce.

The American pattern represented a similar though not entirely
identical compromise. In part, this was through direct emulation.
American reformers visited St Thomas' Hospital and the curriculum of
that school, with its heavily practical emphasis, found its way into a
number of early American training schools.[6] The pattern of student
nurses spending most of their time as ward workers was repeated and
the use of doctors as teachers of nurses again figures large. At Bellevue
Hospital in New York, for example, a training school for nurses was
formally opened in 1873. A small number of wards participated in the
new schemes and only later, as the economics of it were shown to be
viable, was the number extended. As in Britain, the candidates rotated
through the wards, both serving as workers and being taught. The
programme, however, was from the outset for a two-year period; in the
second year students, where possible, were to be promoted to positions
of responsibility, as head nurses, etc. There, as elsewhere, the hospital
came to be staffed almost entirely by trainees.[7]

That this was in some ways a similar sort of compromise is
apparent from a consideration of the school associated with the Johns
Hopkins Hospital in Baltimore.[8] The first superintendent, Miss Hampton,
had begun her working life as a teacher in Canada and her interest in
pedagogy had already borne fruit in her time at the Illinois Training
School where she had introduced a graded system of instruction and
class work and had pioneered a scheme of affiliation whereby students
gained experience in types of nursing not available at the main school.
She was, it would seem, supported in these educational aims by the
medical superintendent who had toured other hospitals in the USA
prior to the establishment of nurse training at Hopkins and had
recommended, among other things, careful attention to the intellectual
part of the training of the nurse. Favourable as these omens seemed to
be for an educational emphasis in the nursing school, it seems that Miss
Hampton was still constrained to follow much of the prevailing pattern.
In four years, to be sure, she had managed to secure a substantial
number of lectures from the medical staff, she had appointed an

assistant superintendent to concern herself with first-year instruction
and she had started a Nurses' Journal Club to study the emerging
periodical literature. Yet her first annual report talks of changes in the
pupils' programme to take account of the needs of the hospital; their
day was a full twelve hours and, inexperienced as they were, they were
often required to assume full responsibility for a ward. Miss Hampton
admitted that the arrangements severely taxed the capacity and
strength of the pupils, leaving them no time for collateral reading.
Changes were secured but often at the price of agreeing to additional
service commitments. Even here, then, under especially favourable
circumstances, the student labour system was in operation.

It is worth underlining how few trained nurses there were in the
American hospitals. The seniority system provided head nurses from
amongst the trainees themselves. On completion of their two-, later
three-year course, these young women would look for nursing work in
the community, free from any contractual obligations to the hospital or
school. The American image of the trained nurse was thus of the
individualistic, independent entrepreneur; the British image was rather
of the faithful employee, with traditional loyalties to her hospital, her
school and her matron.

Different Battles, Different Arenas

The early phase of local effort and initiative to establish training schools
met with growing enthusiasm and on both sides of the Atlantic more
and more hospitals opened nurse training schools.[9] But this was neither
a recognition of the value of the trained nurse nor an acceptance of the
need for provision of training. Rather, it was a pragmatic welcome for a
trainee who made few demands either on the budget of the hospital or
on the existing social relations within it. Both sets of nursing leaders
fought for change; interestingly, neither condemned outright the plight
of the trainee or demanded specialised educational resources
independent of service needs. In each case the battle was fought around
themes of 'better standards' or 'recognition', though what these meant
differed sharply in the two contexts.

In Britain after 1860, application to a hospital with a school was not
the only route to becoming a 'trained nurse'. For one thing, there was a
whole host of local nursing associations, groups of perhaps half a dozen
or so nurses who would band together to provide home nursing in a
particular locality and who would recruit one or more probationers.

For another thing, there were the training associations, independent bodies set up specifically to provide a training, which then negotiated with voluntary hospitals to provide clinical work.[10] And thirdly, there were the various workhouse nursing associations. In London, for example, as Rosemary White points out, the Association for Promoting Trained Nursing in Workhouses was by 1885 paying for the training of nurses and afterwards placing them in workhouse nursing posts; and in Liverpool, the Northern Workhouse Nursing Association formed in 1891 fulfilled a similar role. Questions of criteria for recruitment, of conditions for approval of hospitals as Schools of Certification, were quite clearly being raised in these contexts, and indeed there were some, in the workhouse nursing area, who had by 1902 begun to think about and make suggestions for a nationwide nursing service and a regularised set of conditions for training.[11]

These institutionalised arrangements have been neglected in a history which concentrates upon personalities and politics. We are much more familiar with the 'battle for registration', with the campaigning of the British Nurses' Association, with the way in which Florence Nightingale trounced it in its aims of setting up a register of all qualified nurses and making itself the body which would inspect and approve training schools. There is room for much more study of what Dean and Bolton (elsewhere in this volume) would call a 'discourse' concerning the regulation of training, and of the way in which that discourse at first envisaged and endorsed the regulation of training not just by hospitals, but by voluntary associations of various sorts and by groups wholly comprised of nurses. In the end, of course, that discourse centred around state regulation – a procedure for licensing nurses broadly comparable to that already found acceptable for other occupational groups, notably, in the health field, doctors and midwives.

The General Nursing Council (GNC) was set up in 1919. It was a body charged with the duty of maintaining a register of all trained nurses and determining the conditions for entry to it; it was not, however, a body with the responsibility and resources to organise nurse education *per se.*[12] The GNC, the powers of which were set out in outline form only in the legislation of 1919, was soon to learn what little say it had in the conduct of nurse education. It was overridden by the minister when it wished to determine a lower bed limit for hospitals wishing to be training schools. It was denied the right to issue a training syllabus, though an examination syllabus was in order. It had no resources to inspect schools. It had no powers to close schools or to bring sanctions to bear on schools which did not apply for GNC

approval. It could not stop other bodies from continuing to offer a
nurse training. It had no budget to provide schools with equipment,
facilities or staff or to give grants to trainees. It set no entrance test and
the hospitals continued to recruit whomsoever they pleased as
probationers. What the GNC did do was to devise and administer an
examination and admit names of those who passed on to the register.

The GNC was in an unenviable position. It had to decide on how to
assimilate existing nurses onto the register and how to conduct an
election for places on the Council. It had to devise and implement an
examination procedure. Moreover, it had to do these things in the face
of a suspicious Parliament, disagreement in its own ranks and vigilant
but disparate sets of rank-and-file interests. It was in no way the
moment to sit back and reflect that a new body, superimposed on an
old compromise, was likely to face all the blame for the old
inadequacies. Instead of a major battle, there were small skirmishes
and some successes. The GNC, as time went on, gained a few inspectors,
won a ruling for a minimum number of beds for training, and for a
brief period in the late 1930s also managed to impose an entrance test
on candidates. But by and large the GNC had had no new resources and
no sanctions to apply to the old scheme of nurse education.[13]

In the USA in the same period, the struggles of nurses were
differently constituted and differently perceived. In the first place, and
following the American pattern of political practice, the battle for
recognition of training was conducted at a local level, state by individual
state. Nurses were there with other occupational groups in a battle for
state licensing. What they achieved in the way of legislation was often
minimal; it depended on the forces ranged against them — sometimes
commercial schools, sometimes medical interests, sometimes the
exclusion of women as women from public office, sometimes all of
these and more.[14] Many of the Nurse Practice Acts did not actually
divert resources towards nurse education in any clear way any more
than did the British legislation. But the laws were varied and they were
amendable. State nurses' associations saw achievements elsewhere as a
spur to their own demands and Nurse Practice Acts were constantly
challenged and amended, and indeed continue to be so, up to the
present day.

In the second place, there was what the nurse leaders called an
'educational movement' which they saw as additional to and perhaps
even more important than state registration *per se*. As early as 1893
nursing heads of hospitals had banded together to form a Society of
School Superintendents (later to become the broader-based National

League for Nursing Education). This body served to reinforce a teaching identity via its multiple and energetic activities. Early in its life, for example, it discussed a three-year curriculum and started to outline its content. Later this was to result in the publication of curriculum guides. Studies were carried out of working hours, and schemes and campaigns to limit hours ensued. An education sub-committee was set up and explored ways and means of further training for superintendents themselves.

All of this was largely an indirect effort to raise standards. The Society acted as a resource centre; it provided ideas, support and encouragement from amongst its own numbers. It did not seek closure of substandard schools or the uniform implementation of any curriculum or organisation. It encouraged the already good to become better by dint of more effort, it concentrated on maxima not minima, trying, as it were, to raise the ceiling not the floor. In short, it stressed self-improvement.[15]

Nurses were aided in their efforts at self-improvement and upgrading by the special nature of the American educational system which has always operated in a more 'open' way than the British. Routes to learning are more numerous and more varied; the individual is encouraged to build a mixture of courses suitable for her/his own advancement and flexible entry and multiple choice reflect this. In higher education rigid distinctions between the pure and applied are not drawn and vocational and even practical courses appear as legitimate options in the curriculum. American universities in the inter-war period put on courses for journalists and social workers, and covered librarianship, hospital management, gymnastics and even clogdancing. They catered, as one critical commentator put it, to 'fleeting, transient and immediate needs'.[16]

This made possible a number of developments in nursing education which were unthinkable within the British framework. In 1899, fired by enthusiasm in the Superintendents' Society, its members interviewed the Dean of Teachers College in New York and persuaded him that he should approve a course in hospital economics. The society found the funds, approved the candidates and provided the lecturers from its own ranks. Members worked to build an endowment and it was not until seven years later that some College funding was actually made available.[17] Two years before this development, the University of Texas had integrated a hospital school into its medical department and in 1910 the University of Minnesota began a full pre-registration nursing course, granting a special professional degree. By 1923 there were at least another seven universities giving such a degree; furthermore, 13 universities and three colleges had initiated programmes of four or five years leading to both a college degree and a nursing diploma. At a post-registration level there were 20 schools or courses in public health nursing in the year 1919–20. Whereas prior to 1917 all except the Teachers College course had been started by visiting nurses' associations or other public health organisations, the later courses were associated with universities.[18]

We should not get carried away by all this activity. In the first place, it covered a very small proportion of the total amount of nurse training. Most nurses continued to train in hospitals and to get hospital diplomas. In the second place, college programmes, where they did exist, were usually run on a shoestring too. Both of these points will be elaborated in the section below. For the moment we can observe that both contemporary British and contemporary American nurses would probably have recognised the truth of this (American) insider's comment:

> The big question was not how much the probationer understood about her duties but how much she could get done in a ten hour day and how fast she could learn to take a full share of the work of the hospital ward.[19]

A Strikingly Different Debate

The early 1920s were not easy years for British nurses; they had secured a Registration Act but, as Abel-Smith has shown so clearly, that marked not an end, but a new beginning to their struggle. Disagreements were aired with an embarrassing degree of publicity.[20] No sooner had the examination system got under way (with, as we have seen, little change in the educational institutions) than a new and urgent debate began to be voiced concerning staff shortage in the hospitals. Nurses, including, of course, trainee nurses, were the major hospital labour force and it was their practices which came under scrutiny. The nurse education problem and the nurse manpower problem continued to be interlinked in the new era of shortage in the minds of outside observers and of nurses themselves. It was an interlinking which, as before, proved intensely detrimental to the cause of nurse education.

Two crucial changes had occurred. One was a growing demand for hospital care and a deepening financial crisis for the voluntary hospitals. The other was that there were new and different employment opportunities for women. The hospitals wanted more nurses at the very moment when they could not improve conditions to attract them. This was part of the crisis which was eventually to lead to the NHS — but, at the time, it was the nurses themselves who took the blame.

Accusations came first from the doctors. *The Lancet*, as it had done on previous occasions, seized the opportunity to inquire into the nature of the contemporary malaise. A commission was set up 'to enquire into the reasons for the shortage of candidates, trained and untrained, for nursing the sick in general and special hospitals . . . [and] . . . to offer suggestions . . .'[21] The commissioners deliberately set aside questions to do with alterations in the institutions of nurse education. They were not prepared, for example, to consider university schools, a shorter training or a two-grade structure. It being only twelve years since the Nurses' Act, they felt it was too early to tinker with it. Thus they offered no comment on the responsibilities of the GNC, its resources and the facilities available for teaching in the hospitals, even though it was clear from the critical comments they had received that these latter were few. 'We hear', they said,

> of hospitals with well over 100 nurses in training and only one sister tutor; of others employing sister tutors without special diplomas or any teaching experience; and of some who expect sister tutors to combine the duties of home sister or assistant matron with their educational work.[22]

Indeed, their solution was to simplify the examination syllabus, to clarify its intended scope and to eliminate what they saw as undesirable, direct questions on medicine, surgery and gynaecology — not to add resources for nurse education.

On the vexed question of attracting more recruits *The Lancet* Report made a whole range of suggestions. It advocated shorter hours and better conditions, it suggested ways of dealing with the gap between school leaving and hospital work, it touched on matters such as age of entry, pay, accommodation, food, uniforms, the opening up of administrative careers for nurses and so on. There was much here that nurses themselves could readily accept. But there was another and most important theme. The popularity of nursing as a career would only be restored, they argued, with a modernisation of attitudes amongst the trained nurses themselves. Trained nurses had erected a

system of work organisation which stressed strict discipline, which
placed a value on routine, which gave responsibility on the wards
without trust in the home, which demanded obedience, punctuality and
unswerving loyalty. Ward sisters, they patronisingly opined, 'especially
those who have given their lives to hospital service without administrative promotion, may be intolerant of attempts to induce them to
allow others a discipline less severe than that which they willingly
impose upon themselves'.[23] It was not, then, in the doctors' view, that
the resources for nurse education were inadequate, and that for this
reason training was unattractive; it was rather that the people who ran
it were inadequate. It would not be important to stress this if it had not
caught on as an interpretation of the predicament of the time. But it
did. Not only did it remain unchallenged by the nurses,[24] but it was
importantly endorsed by an official governmental inquiry which
followed.[25] Nurses, apparently, had much to do to put their own house
in order. No one, it seems, argued that high drop-out figures and failure
rates were inevitable when so few resources were allocated to nurse
education, no one pushed the view that nursing service and nurse
education were incompatible goals. These were parts of the initial
compromise and as such they were still, in the late 1930s, entirely
intact.

American nurses, by contrast, carried out their own independent
studies. They came to a conclusion at once more favourable to nurses
themselves and more challenging to the *status quo*. In the event, as we
shall see in the next section, for all their challenging ideas and confident
analyses, the changes they could actually make were minimal. For the
moment, however, we can concentrate on the terms of the debate
itself and on its striking contrasts with that conducted in Britain.

The early 1920s was an exciting time for American nurses. More and
more, the field of public health work was opening up to them. A
campaign was under way with demonstration projects supported by
professionals, by voluntary associations and by federal and local
government funds.[26] The Red Cross, the Rockefeller Foundation, the
Milbank Memorial Fund, the Metropolitan Life Insurance Company
were some of the agencies coming forward with funds; a nursing
division had been set up in the US Public Health Service in 1919; the
Shepard—Towner Act inaugurated an eight-year maternity and infant
care programme which resulted in the first public health nursing
consultants appointed in peacetime to work under governmental
auspices. There was nothing comparable to the early years of the GNC
to demoralise American nurses; indeed, as we have seen, the state-by-

state style of constant legislative amendment kept nurses confidently in the political fray. Furthermore, the very pattern of employment and of education meant, for some at any rate, a lively scepticism as to the viability of the whole system of producing nurses. This point requires some expansion.

Trained nurses did not in the USA, as they did in Britain, find employment in the hospitals. They were to be found, at least until the onset of the Depression, largely in private home nursing and in public health work. A small but increasing number too found employment in college posts, teaching nurses who were qualifying through this route. There was thus the contradiction of a hospital training for community work, and this did not escape the notice of nurses interested in developing training programmes. Adelaide Nutting[27] was one leading American nurse who had long seen this and seen it clearly. In 1901 she was already casting around for models in other occupational groups of how to organise training; in 1905 she was pointing out that a training does and should cost money; by 1908 she was convinced that not all hospitals were fitted to provide a training.[28] Her researches into hours and pay persuaded her that hospitals were closing their eyes to the true costs of nurse training and using students as labour. Training schools, she began to argue, should not be 'charitable institutions' in this way.

When, in 1918, a group of doctors began to suggest that shortages of public health nurses indicated the need for a new non-nurse grade, Miss Nutting was in a strong position to help turn a threat into an opportunity. With Rockefeller Funds an inquiry was mounted; the investigating committee comprised members for the most part in education and public health. It had a social researcher for its secretary. The terms of reference were broadened to cover 'the entire field occupied by the nurse and other workers of related type' and the whole investigation took five years.[29]

Education was needed, the report argued, not just for basic nurses but for hospital superintendents and for public health nurses. The average school fell short of requirements for basic training because of the lack of independent funding, but, given such funding, the consequent improvement in nurse education in the schools would help attract more recruits. To have some university schools was important too, as the 'keystone of the entire arch', furnishing new leaders in teaching and administration. The report, then, not only vindicated the nurses' position on public health work, but thoroughly criticised the hospital schools and laid the blame upon a lack of financial independence. A strong critique of hospital training emerged, in part perhaps through the personal influence of Miss Nutting, and in part perhaps because of the membership composition of the inquiry.[30]

In practice, three endowed schools were set up in the wake of this report. Another consequence, however, was that the nursing organisations got together to carry out their own study. A massive eight-year programme of publicity ensued. It assessed the demand for and the supply of nurses; it asked how successful the present system had been in supplying the right nurses for the right jobs; and it collected information on and elevated the schools themselves.[31]

'Too many yet too few' was one catchphrase of the study. The explosion of training schools had actually meant widespread unemployment amongst trained nurses in 1926 (well before the Depression). There were, the authors argued, 'twin evils of overproduction and undereducation', and these had come about because schools were run as adjuncts to the management of hospitals, not as educational institutions. A massive data collection exercise showed how low the standards of many schools were. The final report was uncompromising in its denunciation of 'conditions which should not be tolerated'. Many of the actual recommendations had been voiced before; what was new was the confident tone. In part, this rested on a new argument, that the recommendations were put forward not in terms of sectional interests, but in the public interest; change would not simply serve nurses — it would serve the community.

American nurses, then, had broken through. They had seen the way in which nurse education had become subordinate to hospital labour and they had found a set of terms in which to condemn it. They had argued that the present system was not in the nurses' interest and, much more importantly, that it was not in the the public interest. This had come at more or less the same chronological moment that British nurses, as we have seen, were acceding in an analysis which put the blame on nurses themselves.

Why this difference of perspective — why this greater confidence among the American nurses? The immediate answer lies in the pattern of institutions available to them. The legislative framework, as we have seen, was conducive to constant change in a way the British centralised system was not; the educational system, again differently constituted, was open to infiltration and provided a vantage point for critics. The pattern of employment too, with its emphasis on private nursing and public health nursing, had helped reveal the inadequacies of hospital training for non-hospital work. These institutions in turn, of course, require study. Why were such arrangements available in American society at this time and why was there a different pattern in Britain? To answer this would take us into a consideration of how economic, political and social forms are deeply intertwined. The point of the present argument, however, is to show that a different matrix of institutions gives different experiences and different opportunities for compromise and struggle for an occupational group such as nurses.

We turn now to the issue of the effects of these contrasting institutional patterns and demands. Did the challenge put forward by the American nurses have any effect? Was the pattern of nurse education significantly altered by the analysis nurses were at pains to spread amongst their own ranks and elsewhere?

The Pattern of Educational Provision

In Britain the provision for nurse education continued to be minimal. This is not surprising in view of the prevailing attitudes to the nurse staffing question outlined above. A sample survey of hospitals carried out in 1930 showed nurses in training to be doing nine to ten hours of routine work per day. Of the hospitals surveyed, little more than a quarter had provided for lectures to be in duty time and hence, for the majority, formal learning was in addition to these long hours on duty. Small hospitals were approved as training schools; in 1938, for example, there were 31 recognised training schools with less than 50 beds. The total number of schools was still increasing, and as far as can be ascertained there was still less than one tutor per recognised general training hospital. Furthermore, there were still hospitals recognised for training by bodies other than the GNC and unapproved hospitals too recruited trainees to solve their staffing problems.[32]

There is an urgent job to be done, if we are better to understand the problems of nurse education today, in exploring in more depth the resources and facilities which were available for nurse training in the 1930s. For these represented the legacy inherited by the NHS. In respect of nurse training (as indeed of other aspects) the NHS did not constitute a revolutionary change. It is possible to argue, and I would contend, that the initial compromise in nurse education was still intact; the student labour system was unchallenged, and the history of the NHS in respect of providing facilities and staff for nurse education continued to be dogged by that compromise without ever addressing it directly.[33]

What, then, of the position in the USA — having uncovered a pattern
of student exploitation by hospital employers, were nurses in any
position to overcome it? The answer, by and large, is no. Later on, in
the immediate post-war period, nurses started to use the mechanism of
accreditation of schools as a sanction, albeit a gentle one and slow in its
operation. Now, in the 1930s, strong as their condemnations were,
these operated still as a kind of shaming strategy. Schools were exhorted
to be better, the nursing associations continued to act as a storehouse
of ideas and energetic nurse leaders put their energy into exemplary
schemes which were implemented in that small number of places where
circumstances were favourable.

Some of the poorer training schools did close in the 1930s. They
closed as training schools because economic distress had cast trained
nurses into the marketplace and these women were prepared to work
for a minimal rate to secure for themselves board and lodging. It made
economic sense, in other words, for hospitals to close their schools. But
poor schools, on the nurses' criteria, certainly remained. In 1951–52,
for example, when a special accreditation procedure was under way,
involving criteria by no means as stringent as some of the schools had
suggested, a mere 18 per cent of over a thousand programmes evaluated
were fully accepted. A study of nursing schools in 1949 revealed a
picture depressingly similar to that which had emerged from the grading
committee's inquiries in 1929 and 1932. To be sure, there had been
changes, but hospital-centred curricula, limited teaching facilities and
small numbers of teaching staff were a familiar pattern[34] and the
overwhelming majority still trained in hospitals rather than colleges.
The journals and associations were setting a pace which few could
follow. As one writer, who has traced in detail efforts to improve
schools in the 1950s, put it: 'the guideposts were so placed that only
the vanguard group of nursing educators could see them directly; they
were barely legible to the lagging majority and were all but invisible to
the stragglers at the rear of the procession'.[35]

A further element which emerged in the 1950s had to do with
collegiate and university programmes. We have already noted how
some of these were set up only by dint of heroic efforts on the part of
nurses themselves. By the 1950s a veritable kaleidoscope of
programmes had emerged, some, perhaps many, of which made
dubious educational sense. Hospital experience might be tacked on to a
collection of courses already on offer in a college to make a degree
programme, the order or mix of components being dictated by
common sense more than anything else. Integration here was more of

an aspiration than a reality. The diploma programmes of the schools and the baccalaureate degree programmes of the colleges were not clearly differentiated. Whether the degree was a post-basic specialisation or an alternative basic course was not clearly thought through and caused further confusion. Whether or not the nurse educators had coherent ideas on these subjects was beside the point; colleges put on courses if they fitted their resource mix and attracted students, and slowly, starting in the early 1950s, the studies conducted through the nursing organisations began to document the chaos which ensued. College programmes *per se* in the American context were not necessarily the answer to all the problems of a nurse education system, though this was a point few appreciated in the 1930s.[36]

The British/American comparison is a salutary one. To be sure, American nurses had developed a much more critical and confident analysis of their own position; they had formulated a clear analysis in the way their British counterparts had not. Yet this made very little difference. In practice, hospitals maintained their schools where these made economic sense. In the US case, where college and university provision was much more open, where vocational courses were countenanced provided they paid their way, these courses too were caught up in an economic logic which overrode strictly educational considerations. In no way, then, did the American pattern mean an unambiguous allocation of resources to nurse education.

Conclusion

Nineteenth-century British nurses made a compromise as far as education and training were concerned. They opted for an 'on the job training', offering their services as staff from the day they entered the hospital gates. The plan had economic advantages and it seemed socially acceptable. It is hard to see how they could have acted otherwise. But the compromise captured minds; it became entrenched as the obvious and appropriate way of staffing the hospitals and training nurses. No one was able to challenge it, not even the nurses themselves. *Nurses forgot their own history*, they acceded in an analysis which presented their members as old fashioned and authoritarian, and their terms and conditions as simply lagging behind those elsewhere.

Nineteenth-century American nurses made a similar sort of compromise. They, too, staffed the hospitals in their student days, but they then left, largely to work on their own account as private nurses or to join public health programmes. Some, given the American emphasis on self-improvement and social mobility and the more open educational structure associated with this, persuaded colleges and universities to train them further and to provide first-level training at that. From these rather different vantage points a critique of the hospital school system emerged. But the critique alone was not sufficiently powerful to demolish that system, nor was it sufficiently encompassing to see that similar kinds of points might also be made against a number of courses in the educational sphere. The American nurse education pattern, in a different way from the British, was none the less also a casualty.

In nurse education, as in many other spheres, Americans and British looked in different directions for salvation. The former turned to the marketplace, to free and open competition, to rugged individualism. When charitable foundations gave them backing, all kinds of innovative programmes emerged — involving things far removed from the normal educational programmes of the local hospitals. Diversity was the keynote. The British have looked and still look to the state for salvation. Nurses petitioned for nationwide recognition and licensing and a single state examination; having achieved that, the state in the 1930s was preparing, albeit hesitantly, to take on a much more interventionist role in planning and regulating nursing manpower. It is interesting to speculate on what might have occurred had these deliberations come to fruition. It would have been difficult to avoid the question of the student labour system. As it was, the war intervened, and in the deliberations about a national health service the issue of the costs of nurse education were obscured. Nurse education entered the NHS with the initial compromise securely intact. Neither state nor marketplace had offered a neutral and disinterested solution to the question of nurse education.

There is a kind of history which insists on viewing change as progress. It documents each 'advance', each 'gain', and attributes it to individuals and to organised groups. Such a history could be written about nurse education. It would deal with the lengthening and changing curriculum and the more stringent requirements of an institution which wished to be a training school; it would catalogue the improving qualifications of those who teach nurses. Such a history has two key limitations. In the first place, it can deal with slow change or no change only as inefficiency, lack of motivation or bumbledom. In the second place, it is consistently blind to the assembled forces which prevent some kinds of change from ever appearing on the agenda.

One advantage of a cross-national comparative history such as this is that it forces us to enlarge the agenda. Why didn't British nurses see the education problem in the way that American nurses did and vice versa? An adequate answer lies in a much deeper understanding of the economic, political and social structure than I have begun to sketch in here. Once we have that, we will see more clearly how nursing education in different ways has been a casualty to other concerns. Perhaps it still is, but that is another story.

Acknowledgement

This chapter stems from work carried out in 1977—78 with funding from the Social Science Research Council. I should like to record my thanks for comments on a draft to Gail Bolton, Ros Brown, Joan Fretwell and Margot White.

Notes

1. For the purposes of this chapter I am ignoring the complexity of initial specialisation in nurse training and the fact that there is no single 'basic' training in Britain. My remarks should be taken as referring for the most part to training for the general register.
2. The best easily accessible source is still probably the history co-authored by two American nurses, Lavinia Dock and Adelaide Nutting: M. A. Nutting and L. L. Dock, *A History of Nursing*, 2 vols (G. P. Putnam's Sons, New York and London, 1907). Two further volumes with the same title were later added by Dock alone. An abbreviated single-volume version of this work is also available. L. L. Dock and I. M. Stewart, *A Short History of Nursing* (G. P. Putnam's Sons, New York and London, 1938). I am also indebted here and in much of what follows, of course, to the classic work on British nurses: B. Abel-Smith, *A History of the Nursing Profession* (Heinemann, London, 1960).
3. Discussions will be found in most of the standard texts. One which I have found particularly helpful is L. Seymer, *A General History of Nursing* (Faber and Faber, London, 1932), Ch. 9. This is usefully supplemented by the more specialist work, L. Seymer, *Florence Nightingale's Nurses: the Nightingale Training School 1860—1960* (Pitman, London, 1960).
4. Several writers of late have drawn attention to the striking parallels between nurses' hospital roles and the position of women in the Victorian home. See B. Ehrenreich and D. English, *Witches, Midwives and Nurses*, Glass Mountain Pamphlet no. 1 (Compendium, London, 1973); M. Carpenter, 'The New Managerialism and Professionalism in Nursing', in M. Stacey *et al.* (eds), *Health Care and the Division of Labour* (Croom Helm, London, 1977); E. Gamarnikow, 'Sexual Division of Labour: the Case of Nursing', in A. Kuhn and A. Wolpe (eds), *Feminism and Materialism* (Routledge and Kegan Paul, London, 1978).
5. See Seymer, *Florence Nightingale's Nurses*.
6. This was true for Bellevue (see note 7), also for training schools in Boston,

New Haven and Illinois. Emissaries in some cases were sent to see Florence
Nightingale personally; elsewhere new schools relied on information previously
secured by longer-established ones.

7. See D. Giles, *A Candle in her Hand: a story of the Nursing Schools of
Bellevue Hospital* (Putnam, New York, 1949).

8. The account which follows is drawn from E. Johns and B. Pfefferkorn, *The
Johns Hopkins Hospital School of Nursing 1889–1949* (The Johns Hopkins Press,
Baltimore, 1954).

9. It is no easy matter to plot exact numbers of schools and to ensure
comparability. The American data are fuller, one source for example showing 15
schools in 1880, 432 in 1900, 1,755 in 1920. US Bureau of the Census, *Historical
Statistics of the United States, Colonial Times to 1970* (Government Printing
Office, Washington, 1975). The British material is more sparse and difficult to
interpret, but my own researches suggest that the number of schools was still
increasing between 1930 and 1946.

10. Neither the local nursing associations nor the training associations have
received much attention from nursing historians. Even Abel-Smith, *Nursing
Profession*, does not cover them very fully. The extent of local nursing association
activity is indicated in the various versions and editions of Burdett's guide to
training schools. See, for example, Sir H. Burdett, *Burdett's Official Nursing
Directory 1898* (The Scientific Press, London, 1898). Reference to the early
history of the London Training School for Nurses (later the British Nursing
Association) and its short-lived contract with St Mary's Hospital, Paddington,
from 1867, is to be found in Z. Cope, *A Hundred Years of Nursing at St. Mary's
Hospital, Paddington* (Heinemann, London, 1955), Ch. 3. Cope makes clear that
the British Nursing Association (not to be confused with the British Nurses'
Association) was still in action in 1884.

11. I have drawn these specific points from Rosemary White's recent study. In
a particularly interesting chapter of her work she draws attention to schemes for
the regularisation of training and for a poor law nursing service which emanated
from workhouse nursing associations. R. White, *Social Change and the Development of the Nursing Profession: a Study of the Poor Law Nursing Service 1848–
1948* (Henry Kimpton, London, 1978), Ch. 7.

12. The account by Abel-Smith, *Nursing Profession*, of the GNC and of the
battles which preceded and followed it remains unsurpassed. I have made brief
reference to the argument here elsewhere: C. Davies, 'Four Events in Nursing
History: a new Look', *Nursing Times*, 74, 17 (1978).

13. Dock, *History of Nursing*, vol. 3, Ch. 2.

14. For details see H. Munson, *The Story of the N.L.N.E.* (W. B. Saunders,
Philadelphia and London, 1934).

15. I have elaborated on the self-improvement strategy and its congruence
with American values in an unpublished paper: C. Davies, 'Professionalising
Strategies as Time- and Culture-Bound: the case of American Nursing circa 1893',
paper read to the BSA Medical Sociology Conference, York, 1978.

16. A. Flexner, *Universities: American, English and German* (Oxford
University Press, New York, 1930), p. 44. For the relevance of these differences to
nursing curricula see C. Davies, 'Curriculum Studies and Institutions: the Case of
Nursing in Britain and the USA' (University of Warwick, mimeo, 1979).

17. For a vivid and lively account of nursing education programmes at
Teachers College see T. E. Christy, *Cornerstone for Nursing Education* (Teachers
College Press, Columbia University, New York, 1969).

18. This information was collated in the course of the Winslow–Goldmark
inquiry discussed later in the chapter. Committee for the Study of Nursing
Education, *Nursing and Nurse Education in the United States* (Macmillan, New
York, 1923).

19. I. Stewart, 'A Half-Century of Nursing Education', *American Journal of Nursing*, 50 (1950), p. 617. See also I. Stewart, *The Education of Nurses: Historical Foundations and Modern Trends* (Macmillan, New York, 1944).

20. See Abel-Smith, *Nursing Profession*.

21. 'The Lancet Commission on Nursing: Final Report' (*The Lancet*, London, 1932), p. 7.

22. Ibid., para. 235.

23. Ibid., para. 37.

24. It was unchallenged in the sense that no direct refutation or counter-analysis emerged. Indeed, the *Nursing Times* felt it expressed nurses' 'own convictions' and did so 'infinitely better than it has hitherto been in our power to do'. One week later, the same journal was urging its readers to accept with humility the findings of the report. *Nursing Times*, 20 and 27 February 1932. For an analysis of the position of the College of Nursing around the time of these reports and for further affirmation that the problem was seen as a 'shortage' one, see C. Davies, 'Continuities in the Development of Hospital Nursing in Britain', *Journal of Advanced Nursing*, 2 (1977). There is a parallel between the analysis there referring to the continuation of a particular 'initial strategy' in nursing and the analysis here which refers to that strategy in respect of education as a 'compromise'.

25. Ministry of Health and Board of Education, *Inter-Departmental Committee on Nursing Services: Interim Report* (HMSO, London, 1939). The work of this committee came to a halt with the outbreak of war, and its interim report was thus the only one ever issued. This report stressed the pre-eminent importance of the shortage problem; though it was much more cautious, it none the less underlined *The Lancet* Commission's criticisms on the question of nurse discipline. It had harsh things to say about the GNC. For these reasons, I would argue that it contributed to the adverse picture of nurses. Furthermore the report represented an important groping towards a position of greater public responsibility for nursing and greater public control over aspects of nursing.

26. For details see M. M. Roberts, *American Nursing: History and Interpretation* (Macmillan, New York, 1954). Miss Roberts was editor of the *American Journal of Nursing* and draws on the volumes of that journal for her most useful history.

27. Mary Adelaide Nutting joined the first class at the Johns Hopkins Training School (1889). Later she became principal of the school. In 1907, she joined the staff of Teachers College and was the first nurse to hold a full professorship. She was active in the formation and development of the major nursing organisations and published widely. See H. E. Marshall, *Mary Adelaide Nutting: Pioneer of Modern Nursing* (The Johns Hopkins University Press, Baltimore and London, 1972).

28. M. A. Nutting, *A Sound Economic Basis for Schools of Nursing and Other Addresses* (Putnam, New York, 1926).

29. Committee for the Study of Nursing Education, *Nursing and Nurse Education*.

30. The inquiry at first comprised a small group of seven, all of whom were in one way or another associated with the educational programmes of Teachers College. Four of the seven were nurses, six of the seven had taught at Teachers College at one time or another. Professor Winslow, as chairman, was head of the School of Public Health at Yale. See Christy, *Cornerstone*.

31. This study generated a number of separate publications and was widely discussed in the American nursing press. The final report gives details of this activity. Committee on the Grading of Nursing Schools, *Nursing Schools Today and Tomorrow* (the Committee, New York, 1934).

32. These data are drawn from the two inquiries already cited, namely *The*

Lancet Commission and the Athlone Report, supplemented by the very useful material collected in a further government-sponsored study: Ministry of Health *et al.*, *Report of the Working Party on Recruitment and Training of Nurses* (Wood Report) (HMSO, London, 1947). The Wood Report is interesting as an 'oddity'. It was a small group, unorthodox in composition and in some respects it burst through what I have called the 'initial compromise'. It was largely ignored. On this see Davies, 'Continuities'.

33. Here, of course, I am asserting a line of argument, rather than supporting it in detail. My convictions stem from a reading of the annual reports of the GNC (available in published form for the period from 1949) and a consideration of what did and did not change for nurses under the NHS legislation and the Nurses' Act of 1949. The GNC in the post-war period was faced with the old arguments about nursing and with worries about high failure and drop-out rates. There was a strong tendency, I would argue, once again to accept the prevailing analysis of these as the fault of nurses themselves rather than as the fault of a compromising system. Over the years we can trace a series of small concessions slowly gained, but no real challenge mounted to the basis of nurse education.

34. For the picture at around 1930 see Committee on the Grading of Nursing Schools, *Report of the First Grading Study of Nursing Schools* (the Committee, New York, 1930); also, by the same group, *The Second Grading of Nursing Schools* (the Committee, New York, 1933). For information for 1949, consult M. West and C. Hawkins, *Nursing Schools at the Midcentury* (National Committee for the Improvement of Nursing Services, New York, 1950).

35. E. Cunningham, *The Social Improvement Programme of the National League for Nursing 1951–60* (NLN, New York, 1963), pp. 4–5.

36. The study of collegiate nurse education strictly belongs to a later period, but the point about its dubious 'educational' character began to emerge strongly in the study by M. Bridgman of *Collegiate Education for Nursing* (Russell Sage Foundation, New York, 1935).

6 ASYLUM NURSING BEFORE 1914: A CHAPTER IN THE HISTORY OF LABOUR[1]

Mick Carpenter

At first glance, a reader is likely to be fascinated with the wealth of new material offered by Mick Carpenter in this chapter on the terms and conditions and on the regulation of the work of the asylum nurse. But Carpenter is doing much more than presenting us with hitherto unfamiliar facts. His real concern is to tie together the working conditions and work experience of nurses in the asylums with the kinds of aspirations which, in the face of such work experiences, these nurses had. Once this is done, trade unionism comes over, not as an aberrant reaction of a few deviants, but as a normal reaction to specific circumstances of work.

All who would write a 'history from below' suffer because the rank and file leave fewer records than do the elite. But, as we can see in this chapter, much can be achieved by interrogating elite records from a rank-and-file point of view. Furthermore, trade union journals give one part of the rank-and-file point of view, and Carpenter uses them when they become available. This is an early report on aspects of a project, not on nursing history as such, but on trade union history. If it serves to bring psychiatric nursing out of obscurity, we must not forget that there are other specialisms equally deserving of study. Carpenter's remarks early in the chapter about how asylum nursing has been neglected and demeaned could well be considered also in the light of these other specialisms.

—————Ed.

Introduction

The men and women who nurse the mentally disturbed seldom achieve public attention, except as a result of scandal or a case of alleged ill treatment. Public interest in psychiatric nursing, if displayed at all, invariably focuses on the sensational. By contrast, there appears to be an almost insatiable public interest in the lives and work of general nurses, who are invariably idealised as 'angels'. In 1961 Alexander Walk complained of 'the almost complete neglect of mental nursing in current histories whether of nursing or psychiatry'.[2] It is a judgement which still holds. Psychiatric nursing lacks glamour and as a result few historians have been interested.

This chapter pieces together the beginnings of a history of nurses in public asylums during the nineteenth and early twentieth centuries. It claims neither to idealise nor to sensationalise, to portray neither angels

nor rogues, but tries to begin reconstructing an informed account of the
work they did, the difficulties they experienced and the sense they tried
to make of their lives. Though objective, it is not detached. Values do
not 'intrude' — they are an inevitable and indeed necessary part of the
approach of historians to their subject-matter. We should, as Gouldner
advises, seek to be 'reflexive' — that is, not abandon our values but be
self-consciously aware of the extent to which they influence our work.[3]

Nursing historians cannot in most cases be praised for their degree of
self-awareness. Within the dominant empiricist approach are half-buried
value assumptions which need to be prised out and exposed to the light
of day. One of these is that nursing history is the history of general
hospital nursing. Other branches receive scanty, if any, attention. In
this way historians confirm, rather than question, the dominance of
hospital nursing in the constellation of nursing and nursing-linked
occupations. To describe these other occupations we use prefixes:
community, psychiatric, mental handicap and so on. When we say
'nurse', however, everyone knows a general hospital nurse is signified.
They have thus claimed proprietary rights over the title: other groups
can only use it on licence, can only claim to be particular kinds of
nurses, not nurses as such. A reflexive history of nursing would not
simply give equal weight to all branches of the occupation, but try to
explain how and why they came to relate together in such ways. Such a
history has yet to be written. Abel-Smith's account[4] is often regarded
as definitive, yet is overwhelmingly concerned with general hospital
nursing. It, too, magnifies the history of general hospital nursing into
the history of nursing in general.

Empiricist nursing history is also shown to be selective in the frame
of reference it has adopted towards its chosen subject-matter. It has
focused primarily on the politics of reform and the lives and activities
of nursing reformers. Nursing is reified into an occupation which is
'reformed' and attains ever dizzier heights of recognition. Reformers
are portrayed as heroines who led the public battle to glorify the good
name of nursing. In the process, nursing history has mainly glorified the
good name of elite members of the occupation. It is their efforts which
have seemed sufficiently significant to record as history. The daily
work of the rank-and-file nurse at ward level is hardly examined at all,
let alone what she might have thought about her work.

A new history of nursing is required to reconstruct the history of
different ways of *being* a nurse: why the job, the background and
perspectives of those doing it have changed — or remained relatively
constant. In short, history from below, rather than from above. It is

time to put *nurses* into nursing history.

The whole idea of a separate nursing history is itself ideologically loaded. It was born of the nursing reform movement itself, which sought to convince the world that nursing was a special occupation and, therefore, nurses were special kinds of people. An insular nursing history implicitly seeks to stake out the social distance between nurses, other kinds of health workers and the working class in general. Since I reject the world view which tries to place nurses on pedestals, I reject also the idea of a separate history of nursing, simply regarding it as one chapter in the history of labour.

The Wider Background

In any case, a reflexive account must cast its net wider. To understand why psychiatric nursing emerged requires at least some preliminary inquiry as to why asylums were created at a certain stage in human history. We need to explain what Michel Foucault has dubbed as 'that other form of madness, by which men, in a sovereign act of reason, confine their neighbours, and communicate and recognize each other through the renowned language of non-madness'.[5] We should not, in his view, accept the division of the world into mad and sane as 'neutral'. Foucault turns the dominant approach on its head and denies that this division was a sign of growing social and humanistic concern with society's weaker members. He questions the division of human experience into two sides, relegating one side and the other 'as things henceforth external, deaf to all exchange as though dead to one another'.[6] One of the most important factors contributing to this split was the growing importance of 'rationality' in social and economic life. Whether this idea was dependent or independent of other social changes, it led to the emergence of new norms of social behaviour, based increasingly upon contractual rather than customary obligations between people, appropriate to a market economy. Individual self-control emerged as an imperative, regulatory force in an individualistic, competitive society. The work ethic emerged and, alongside it, a belief in the need to curtail and subordinate human expressiveness and sensuality. Closely allied to this was the idea that future gains could only be achieved at the cost of present abnegation.

Other divisions occurred, between mind and body, intellect and animality, civilisation and savagery; and progress became seen as synonymous with the control of one side of human nature — the dangerous side — by the other. Animality was often implied in the emerging notions of madness — a swamping of the conscious, reasoning and civilised side of human nature by its instinctual, dark, unreasoning, animal side, as a result of a loss of self-control. As Sauvages explained: 'The distraction of our mind is the result of our blind surrender to our desires, our incapacity to control or moderate our passions.'[7] In some ways this view of madness was optimistic. If madness were a form of surrender, it could possibly be corrected by a regime which encouraged the re-establishment of self-discipline. Michael Fears has described how such 'therapeutic optimism' emerged from Tuke's work at the Retreat in York.[8] Tuke sought to reproduce in the Retreat the intimacy of family relations, with the lunatic as a dependent child and himself as the authoritative patriarch. Force was to be used as a last resort. Tuke approvingly quoted John Locke's advice that:

> the great secret of education, lies in finding the way to keep the child's spirit easy, active and free; and yet, at the same time to restrain him from many things he has a mind to, and to draw him to things which are uneasy to him.[9]

The aim of 'moral treatment', then, as Tuke advocated it, was towards 'assisting the patient to control himself'. In other words, a less overtly coercive form of control would better lead to the 'internalisation' of the principles of self-control. Segregation of the insane was necessary to reproduce the dependence that characterised the child's position in the family. The physician, William Battie, felt that treatment 'requires the patient's being removed from all objects that act forcibly upon the nerves and excite too lively a perception of things, more especially from such objects as are the known causes of his disorders'.[10] Since these could include 'affecting friends as well as enemies', all visits should be banned, and 'the place of confinement should be at some distance from home'. Within the asylum, every means was to be found to create a sober, orderly and bland environment which did not excite the passions. Battie even frowned on highly seasoned food. Employment, however, was to be encouraged, in things '(if such there be) between pleasure and anxiety'.[11]

Asylum Nursing in Theory

The successful pursuit of 'moral principles' depended on the personal qualities of those caring for the patients, to a much greater extent than with 'medical' forms of therapy such as bleedings and purges. In the Retreat, the small size of the institution enabled the superintendent to be involved in every aspect of institutional life. Tuke argued:

> against very large Institutions, where the number of patients is too great to come under the proper inspection of the Superintendent; and where they are therefore chiefly left to the care and management of keepers, who too frequently possess few of the qualities necessary for their office, unless we consider as such 'Limbs of British oak and nerves of steel'.[12]

Dr John Conolly, the medical superintendent at Hanwell, was one of the first doctors seriously to adopt the principles of moral treatment in a public asylum. He recognised that, if treatment without recourse to bodily restraints were to prove successful, there was need for attendants of sufficient number and quality. For public asylums he advocated one attendant to 15 patients (but much higher rates in private asylums). Conolly's most insistent complaint was that, by the mid-nineteenth century, physicians were often not responsible for the hiring and discharge of attendants, whom he regarded as the most important feature of an asylum's regime:

> The character of particular patients, and of all the patients of a ward, takes its colour from the character of the attendants placed in it. On their being proper or improper instruments — well or ill-trained — well or ill-disciplined — well or ill-cared for — it depends whether many of his patients shall be cured or not cured; whether some shall live or die; whether frightful accidents, an increased mortality, incalculable uneasiness and suffering, and occasional suicides, shall take place or not.[13]

Gaining formal control over matters relating to the hiring, discipline, training and deployment of attendants, often in competition with lay officials, magistrates and committees, was a vital step for superintendents to establish their institutional authority.

The attendant was especially important to the new system of moral restraint because in the larger, public asylums there were not sufficient doctors to supervise every aspect of treatment. Economy required that responsibility be delegated to attendants. Under the system of non-restraint, Foucault argues, the attendant

> advances upon madness deprived of all that could protect him or

make him seem threatening, risking an immediate confrontation without recourse. In fact, though, it is not as a concrete person that he confronts madness but as a reasonable being, invested by that very fact, and before any combat takes place, with the authority that is his for not being mad.[14]

Yet if, as Foucault suggests, the ideal asylum was 'a complicated machine of many parts' by which the madman was confronted by 'Reason', it also was one which sought to observe closely the actions of attendants and nurses. To ensure that they fulfilled their part in the plan, the asylum became a disciplinary force against subordinate staff as well as patients.

The medical authorities articulated an image of the ideal nurse or attendant who possessed qualities equal to his tasks. This was later systematised in the *Handbook for Attendants on the Insane*, first published in 1885 by a group of psychiatrists on behalf of the Medico-Psychological Association and surviving, with revisions, until the mid-twentieth century. In the textbook's view: 'a good attendant knows his own mind, he has attained self-control; he has a grasp of hygiene, bodily and mental, and possesses those moral qualities summed up in *character*' (original emphasis).[15] The *Handbook* lists 'discipline' as the first of the 'varieties of duty' of an attendant, and further elaborates that discipline has two facets: '(1) As it is imposed on the attendant — that is his duty to the asylum and his fellows; (2) As he should impose it on his patients — that is his duty to his patients'.[16] The most important feature of the attendant's role was, however, behaviour by example: 'Attendants . . . should themselves set an example of industry, order, cleanliness, and obedience.'[17]

Direct comparisons were drawn between the asylum and the hospital, with routine, order and discipline seen as analogous to the principles of hygiene which governed the hospital: 'They tend to keep in subjection excitement and disorder, which are as harmful to the mental invalid as microbes are to a patient with a wound or sores.'[18]

Asylum Nursing in Practice: the Triumph of Pessimism

The ideals were themselves more authoritarian than humane, even when suffused with optimism. They were never officially abandoned, but in practice a mood of profound pessimism set in. Madness became increasingly viewed as an irrecoverable state and the role of medicine, particularly from the 1890 Lunacy Acts, was less to cure than to justify the lunatic's exclusion from society with the finality of 'certification'.

As Scull has shown, as the century progressed asylums became much larger and provided convenient dumping grounds for unwanted members of society: 'The asylum's early association with social reform gave a humanitarian gloss to these huge, cheap, more or less overtly custodial dumps where the refuse of humanity was collected together.' Medical control and the official ideology of 'treatment' 'served to legitimate further the custodial warehousing of these, the most difficult and problematic elements of the disreputable poor'.[19]

Urbanisation and the development of a market economy disrupted traditional means of support. In addition, the establishment feared the 'seething mass', expressed most clearly perhaps in the concept of 'contagion' which, as Pearson has suggested, was a fear of 'political contamination . . . over and above a simple health hazard'.[20] It was a fear of the 'dangerous classes' whose lack of industry, licentiousness and unruliness threatened to engulf other sections of society.

The Victorians built sewers and instituted other public health measures to deal with the threat of physical contagion. But as Pearson has also pointed out, the notion of the sewer had a much wider currency than this. Quoting contemporary sources, he shows that:

Sewage and drains were guiding metaphors for those who depicted the deviants of this time. 'Foul wretches' and 'moral filth' lay heaped in 'stagnant pools' about the streets. When they moved they were seen to 'ooze' in a great 'tide'.[21]

In their way, asylums were like sewers, designed to cleanse cities of 'moral' filth, unobtrusively removing it to a distant place where its threat to decent society could be contained.

This helps to explain the paradox of why Victorians seemed prepared to spend vast sums of money to build and maintain asylums, yet claimed above all to be motivated by economy. The concern was real enough, within a perspective which assumed the necessity of exclusion and viewed prospects of recovery in pessimistic terms. The chief criterion of institutional success was not discharge or recovery rates, but keeping the average weekly cost of maintenance for a pauper lunatic as low as possible.

One such means was the widespread utilisation of patient labour. The latter half of the nineteenth century saw the rapid development of 'asylum industries', often of amazing diversity. These had a profound effect upon the relationships between staff and patients. While the duties of some nurses and attendants were confined to what would normally be described as 'nursing care' tending 'refractory' and debilitated patients, or surveillance of those patients taking exercise on airing courts, others spent much of the time supervising the work of patients. This mirrored the wider division of labour in society: male inmates engaged in a wide diversity of trades and pursuits. For example, at Prestwich Asylum, during 1857, 158 out of 248 male patients were engaged in various trades, including working on the farm, assisting the asylum joiner, engineer, plumber and painter, tailor, upholsterer and baker. Others assisted in cleaning wards and one was engaged in brewing. On the female side, 183 out of 260 patients were supervised in a more limited number of activities: cleaning wards, working in the laundry, knitting and sewing, and picking flocks.[22] Those who were able were therefore expected to contribute to their upkeep by working. Responsible work (such as the laundry for women, the workshops for men) was sometimes a stepping stone to freedom. In many asylums, however, it encouraged medical superintendents to hang on to their most able workers, rewarding them with only a few minor privileges.

Therapeutic pessimism affected the development of asylum nursing in other ways. Earlier in the century, some optimistic superintendents managed to persuade economy-minded committees, concerned about the charge to the rates, to finance improvements. Thus, in the 1830s, some doctors instituted experimental training schemes for attendants. But it was not until the 1890s that the Medico-Psychological Association (the forerunner of today's Royal College of Psychiatrists) began to introduce certificated training on a national scale. Even then, it was many years before training was universal and certificates became a compulsory requirement for applicants for higher posts.

Not surprisingly, staffing ratios were at a minimum consistent with maintaining order. The rulebooks issued to attendants often make clear that order and security were uppermost in the authorities' minds. For example, that of Wiltshire County Asylum for 1882 states:

The points requiring particular attention from the Attendants in the management of their Patients are:
1. Cleanliness and dress.
2. The distribution of food at mealtimes.
3. Exercise in the open air.

4. Occupation.
5. General quietness and good conduct.
6. Amusement.
7. Attention to the calls of Nature, on which all cleanliness and
   health depend.[23]

There is little here regarding moral treatment. Security also occupied a
good deal of space in all rulebooks: care of keys, tools and cutlery. The
London County Asylum's rulebook specified that: 'Attendants and
workmen shall see that all ladders, steps, or other things used by them,
which may enable patients to escape . . . are carefully guarded, and
directly the work is performed, removed out of their reach.'[24]

There were, in fact, relatively few escapes from asylums. For
example, the Escapes Book of Lancaster Asylum in the 18 years from
July 1895 to September 1913 shows that there were only 186 escape
attempts and some of these were repeated offenders. Interestingly, men
were nearly four times as likely as women to make escape attempts. By
law, those who survived recapture for 14 days could not afterwards be
taken back without being recertified.

The result of these developments has led Hunter to claim, perhaps a
shade romantically, that by the end of the nineteenth century the 'fall
of mental nursing' had taken place. Although 'mechanical constraints'
like straightjackets had been abolished, 'chemical constraints' were
taking their place with not dissimilar effects. Yet in his view nursing is
the opposite of 'constraint' and requires favourable staffing ratios in
order that the nurse might 'counter alienation by sustained, kindly,
human understanding and contact'.[25]

The Material Conditions of Asylum Work

Since they sought economy in all things, and regarded the asylum as a
necessary but unproductive burden on the rates, it would be unrealistic
to expect asylum authorities to be generous employers of labour. Thus,
for example, the Wages Book of Lancaster County Asylum shows that
for the year 1887 the highest-paid attendant, one John Stavely,
received £40 and the lowest-paid, R. S. Farrer, £28 a year. The highest-
paid day nurses, like Mary and Agnes Denny, received £22 a year,
while Alice Hayes apparently only merited £16. Reliable wage data for
this period are difficult to obtain but a few comparisons can be made.
Constables in 1886 achieved a considerable improvement in pay which

reached around £75 a year after eight years.[26] Even taking into account payments in kind received by asylum workers, a considerable differential existed. In this respect, agricultural workers, whose wages were among the lowest, are more directly comparable. In 1877 the average wages for an ordinary labourer in England and Wales were approximately £37 a year.[27] This can be compared to the wage rates of a skilled engineering fitter in Manchester in 1871, which were over £83 a year.[28] A Lancashire woman weaver in 1886 could expect a rate of wages amounting to approximately £47 a year.[29] A trained general nurse in a London hospital could, around this time, expect to earn an initial salary of about £26 a year, plus payments in kind which one author estimates to be worth around £11 a year.[30] Domestic servants' wages varied, of course, according to the household, but Charles Booth and Jessie Argyle estimated the average as £18 a year plus allowances.[31] In short, asylum nurses' and attendants' wages were close to the bottom of the league. For men, the most comparable wages were those of agricultural labourers; for women, those of domestic servants.

Another area where asylum work often compared unfavourably with other forms of employment was in hours of work. In the last quarter of the nineteenth century, considerable pressure was mounted within the labour movement to achieve reductions in the working week. Legislation, by the late 1870s, restricted the number of hours worked by women in manufacturing industries to ten hours a day. Unionised male employees were able to use more traditional means of pressure. By 1876 the working week was down to 51 hours for engineers, 54 for iron-founders and 48½ for carpenters.[32] Where neither legislative protection nor union strength existed, hours of work continued to be excessively long well into the twentieth century. Public and professional employment was not covered by limitation of hours provisions in Factory Acts, nor were agriculture or domestic service, the most comparable employments. Hours of work, therefore, remained long, even by the standards of the time. According to Conolly: 'The duties of an attendant in an asylum begin early in the morning, are incessant during the day, and end late.'[33] Conolly details the routine of the attendant's working day: rising at 6 a.m. to get patients ready for the day and to serve breakfast, then cleaning out the wards after patients had been sorted out to their various destinations, after which those who were sick were prepared for medical visits. At every moment during the daytime an appropriate task presented: at eleven o'clock patients were to be exercised in the open air, at one o'clock returned for dinner, at five or six o'clock conducted to chapel for evening service, at eight o'clock to bed. At Hanwell Asylum in the 1840s, the attendants sent in their evening reports to the medical officers and were free until six the next morning. This was a liberal regime: in many asylums the day continued to ten o'clock, and staff slept in rooms adjacent to the wards to be on hand at night. At Hanwell, two attendants took it in turns to sit up after a day's shift, but gradually in many asylums full-time night watches were introduced.[34] Yet 'sleeping in' was still in practice in British mental hospitals in the 1930s.

How little things had improved from the 1840s can be seen by the survey of 31 mental hospitals conducted by the National Asylum Workers' Union in 1912, as part of their (unsuccessful) agitation for legal reductions in hours. With two exceptions, the working week for men and women was found to be in excess of 70 hours a week, exclusive of mealtimes, and in some cases more than 80 or even 90 hours a week. A number of justifications were made by asylum authorities to a House of Commons Select Committee set up in 1911 to investigate asylum employees' conditions of employment. It was sometimes suggested that a shorter day would interrupt continuity of patient care, necessitating a three-shift rather than a two-shift day. Some medical superintendents admitted that hours were long but claimed the duties were often light: 'included in this [number of hours] is time for dressing, and tidying bedroom, also time spent in playing games, cricket and football for the attendants, and stoolball for the nurses – both practice and matches – often without patients'. A Dr Cassidy, the medical superintendent of Lancaster Asylum, went even further and told the committee that one day off a month was enough and positively beneficial to staff: 'I think the effect of too much leave, too much freedom, too many hours off duty, would be distinctly demoralizing, especially to the formal staff.'[35] The effect of long hours, living-in and geographical isolation was to exclude staff from participation in a wider society, to almost the same degree as inmates.

This is not to suggest that there were no pressures to improve wages and conditions during the nineteenth century. The Commissioners in Lunacy in 1859 specifically linked the poor remuneration received by attendants with the complaints of ill treatment made by patients when they visited individual asylums, and sometimes recommended increases.

The development of incremental scales and the emergence of a graded hierarchy among the attendant and nursing labour force probably had much to do with the need to motivate and retain nursing staff, as well as the need to co-ordinate even larger and more complex institutions. Management also began to make posts pensionable and, as in agriculture, to provide low-cost housing which would induce male staff, in particular, to stay on at the asylum. Section 280 of the Lunacy Act 1890 permitted asylums to grant pensions to staff but, owing to pressure from county and county borough councils, who were worried at the expense, this was left to the discretion of authorities, as it had been under an earlier Act of 1853.

The *Medical Press and Circular* in 1900 expressed the view that:

> There is no doubt that the asylum service has been looked down upon in the past as worse and more degrading than the lowest menial service. There was a time when a policeman was looked down upon as exercising an office worse than contemptible. If there could possibly be a degree lower it was filled in olden times, and even in recent times, by the asylum attendant . . .[36]

What had made the difference, according to the author, were pensions, which had served to raise the status of many forms of public service. For example, their benefit in the prison service 'is proved by the low percentage of changes in that service, that a pension is assured for good and faithful service'.[37] Yet in the asylum service they were still not obligatory. The issue was not settled until 1909. The 1909 Asylum Officers' Superannuation Act brought in compulsory but (in line with the Liberal Government's philosophy) contributory pensions. This meant an effective wage cut for those who had been receiving non-contributory discretionary pensions. The furore which this caused led to disillusionment with the Asylum Workers' Association, the professional association which had sponsored legislation, and to its eventual replacement by a trade union, the National Asylum Workers' Union.[38]

The Class Background of Asylum Workers

Given the low wages, long hours and poor conditions, widespread fears that sustained contact with the insane was contaminating, and the increasing general prosperity, it is not surprising that asylum work was often regarded as an occupation of last resort. Dr Browne in 1837 described attendants as 'the unemployed of other professions . . . if they possess physical strength and a tolerable reputation for sobriety, it is enough; and the latter quality is frequently dispensed with'.[39] Medical superintendents often took those they could get: on the male side, ex-servicemen and policemen, whose pensions made them less reluctant to accept low wages; otherwise, especially in rural areas, they competed in the market for farm labourers.

Most authorities set fairly modest ideals for recruitment. Henry Burdett, for example, noted in 1891 that:

> It is the general feeling that no attempt should be made to get ladies and gentlemen, i.e. persons with gentle upbringing, as attendants, because they would never be induced to perform many of the duties required of an attendant in a pauper asylum, and they would be out of sympathy with the tastes of the patients. Even in asylums for the better class of patients the duties of attendants must often comprise many details of a menial character.[40]

According to Dr Conolly, 'The best attendants, both male and female, are to be found in the class of persons who are qualified to be upper servants.'[41] The most important quality was considered to be 'benevolence' combined with a 'moderate share of understanding' which he believed could be purchased by means of 'a fair remuneration and prospect of comfort'.

The ideal recruit was, therefore, a member of the 'respectable' rather than 'rough' section of the working class. The problem was that, on the whole, pay and prospects were not sufficiently attractive to secure their services. Given the emphasis on order, it is also hardly surprising that in practice strength was often prized above benevolence. The tendency, as Conolly in particular was aware, was for staff to be recruited from 'the dangerous classes of society'. In other words, they came from the same sections of society as the patients and often exhibited the same kind of unruly personal behaviour which was then believed to contribute to insanity.

However, by no means all authorities were agreed that the main problem was the lack of material inducements and rewards. W. A. F. Browne, a Commissioner for Lunacy in Scotland, commented disparagingly on the recommendations of the 1859 Report of the English Commissioners in Lunacy to increase pay: 'Such a process might secure better cooks or coachmen, but it is doubtful whether you can buy good tempers and tact and discretion.'[42] Instead, he favoured an attempt to recruit those motivated by vocational ideals, who would view asylum work as 'a calling'. The model was, of course, general nursing, which had succeeded in attracting considerable numbers of the better class of women, desperate to escape from stultifying drawing rooms and prepared to work for low economic rewards and to make a virtue of long hours.

Nightingale herself showed no desire to include asylums within the scope of nursing reform. The links with general nursing did not occur until later. Browne himself felt that it was only the rare individual male attendant who would be likely to be motivated by high ideals of service. Yet perhaps the possibility of attracting greater numbers of women suitably motivated to asylum employment might stand greater prospects of success. Dr Greene, the medical superintendent of Berry Wood Asylum, Northampton, boasted in a public lecture to the Royal British Nurses' Association: 'I have engaged as nurses . . . daughters of military officers, clergymen, lawyers, and many others connected with the liberal professions; governesses, pupil-teachers, farmers' daughters, etc.' He then admitted that many others were of 'the higher domestic servant type' and complained that:

> I fear . . . that the asylum nurse is rather looked down upon in some places, as if she belonged to an inferior order of the nursing profession . . . Certainly, it is true that as yet asylum nursing has not commonly attracted women from the higher classes of society, whereas the hospital has quite often supplied the essential attraction, whatever it may be.[43]

At Berry Wood, training courses were introduced only for female staff in an attempt to attract 'better' recruits. Some authorities also attempted to woo trained staff from general hospitals. This was pioneered in Scottish asylums by Dr Robertson, who reminisced in 1918:

> I induced the first hospital nurses to enter the wards of an Asylum in the year 1895. The prestige of the Asylum service was then so low that it took nearly a year before I could get a single candidate. Two others came shortly afterwards. All three became Matrons of Asylums within three years, and after that candidates became numerous.[44]

The prospect of a rapid rise to a position of rank therefore provided the attraction. In the early days of nursing reform, Nightingale trained nurses had risen rapidly to positions of rank as matrons in hospitals throughout Great Britain and the Empire. These very rapid rates of upward mobility could not be sustained indefinitely, and asylum posts provided an important outlet for the next generation of high flyers.

By 1914, nursing on the female sides of asylums had become a recognised part of the nursing universe. Attempts to extend female nursing, partly for economic reasons, to male sides proved unsuccessful outside Scotland. The main resistance came from male attendants, who saw it as a means of replacing them with cheaper labour. They also resented what they largely regarded as 'general hospital snobs'. Robertson and others hoped that competition from general trained nurses would induce asylum nurses to seek general training in order to qualify themselves for matrons' and assistant matrons' posts. In 1914, an influential book, written as a guide to women on the threshold of careers, advised that:

> Mental nursing as a profession for educated women has much to recommend. It is of absorbing interest to those of a sympathetic nature and of a scientific turn of mind, and it develops all the finer qualities of self-control, patience, tact, and commonsense.[45]

It also pointed to drawbacks: staffing ratios which did not permit individual attention, inadequate social facilities for nurses in their off-duty hours and requirements of considerable devotion. Above all, it advised intending asylum nurses to do general training first.

Discipline and Control in Theory and Practice

Since the search for the self-motivated nurse proved largely unsuccessful, the authorities inevitably fell back upon external controls. Asylums became what Gouldner has called 'punishment-centred' bureaucracies.[46] Long books of rules were issued to staff, supposedly covering every significant eventuality. In addition, some aspects of their behaviour were circumscribed by law, in a way which would have been regarded as unthinkable for general nurses.

Sections 322—24 of the Lunacy Act 1890 made ill treatment or neglect of patients, helping patients to escape or having sexual relations punishable offences. However, it was largely through the rulebooks of individual asylums that staff lives were governed. Staff were often asked to sign 'Obligation Forms' which, as at the Middlesex Asylum, Napsbury, gave the medical superintendent considerable latitude:

> I acknowledge the right of the Superintendent to suspend me

without warning for any acts of unkindness, harshness or insolence, violence to patients, disobedience of elders, transgression of rules or negligence; also for intemperance or immorality, whether occurring within or without the asylum boundaries; in any of which cases the wages due to me will be paid only up to the day of suspension.[47]

Through such means the power of the medical superintendent extended in principle to every area of the staff's working and non-working lives. In some areas, notably London, the superintendent's power was, by the end of the nineteenth century, partly exercised in conjunction with visiting committees. Typically, however, the medical superintendent had the power immediately to dismiss or suspend any nurse or attendant, and visiting committees simply rubber-stamped his decision. In many asylums a complex system of penalties existed. For example, at the Metropolitan Asylums' Board asylums, lateness was punished by a scale of fines ranging from 6d to 2s 6d. Failure to turn a light off at the proper time led to a fine 'not exceeding 6d'. If an attendant did not wear his chain with keys attached, he was fined up to 5s, and a lost key brought a fine of 10s.[48] The latter was fairly lenient, for in many asylums it warranted dismissal. When patients escaped, it was usual for attendants to be asked to pay costs of recapture, which sometimes included a reward to the police constable.

Nearly all rulebooks warned of the danger of gossiping about asylum affairs when outside its bounds, and warned staff that on no account should they carry letters to the outside for patients. Most covered the rules for restraint, seclusion, feeding of patients and maintaining their personal appearance.

Discipline was often harsh and arbitrary. For example, at Lancaster Asylum in 1892, two attendants, one with nearly three years' and one with nearly two years' service, were discharged 'for sitting up playing cards'. Fanny Walker, a housemaid with nearly three years' service, was dismissed in the same year,'for carelessly leaving a door open'.[49] Many asylums had rules regulating marriages between staff (rules which were still in operation well into the twentieth century). Often marriage was sanctioned only with the express approval of the medical superintendent. Intermarriages between male and female staff were particularly frowned upon, and male and female sides were strictly segregated.

The mere existence of strict rules does not of itself, however, guarantee unfaltering adherence to them. Certain rules probably were enforced strictly – particularly those regarding security. However, the means for ensuring total compliance did not exist. As Scull has suggested, medical superintendents retreated from the wards to become 'insulated from the reality of asylum existence'.[50] The day-to-day supervision of attendants was left to assistant medical officers, who were not only few in number but were dependent on the reports of attendants with regard to treatment. Scheff, in a study of an American mental hospital in the 1950s, reached a conclusion that had been true for many years previously: the role that attendants acted as gatekeepers between inmates and doctors gave them enormous potential power, for failure to perform it would overwhelm the medical staff with work.[51] Thus, in many instances, though doctors 'ordered' treatment for individual patients, it must often have been at the behest of attendants. One such doctor described his experience of this process during the First World War:

> The chief cause of the difficulty, of course, was the large number of patients for which each Medical Officer was responsible. I had three hundred and fifty, on an average, under my charge alone . . . It was impossible to bear in mind the individual condition of all these patients.[52]

The doctor had little option in most cases but to follow the advice of attendants. Effectively, attendants and nurses ran the asylums. Dr Charles Mercier, himself a medical superintendent, honestly admitted that:

> The attendants are the backbone of a lunatic asylum . . . To the comfort of ninety nine out of a hundred patients in the asylum the removal and replacement of the Medical Superintendent is a matter of no moment all in comparison with the removal or replacement of the attendant who has immediate charge of them.[53]

Perhaps the existence of long rulebooks served to reassure authorities that they were still in command. Perhaps also it could allow them formally to state that asylums were 'hospitals' for the treatment and cure of the insane, and assert a view that staff should act in accordance with these ideals. After all, it cost nothing to say such things.

The Roots of Unrest

Some of the hesitant moves towards improvements in staff conditions from the 1890s were made in the awareness that unrest was seething —

and not always beneath the surface. For example, the attendants of
Bodmin Asylum petitioned the visiting committee over a plan to extend
the pensionable age from 50 to 55 years. Among their complaints were
the following:

1) The small amount of remuneration we receive compared with the
   length of time we are confined within this institution.
2) The home comforts we have to sacrifice compared with other
   spheres of life.
3) The dangers that we are daily subjected to.
4) The unhealthy, disagreeable, injurious things we have to contend
   with daily.[54]

They complained also that in a number of cases staff had been so
'broken' by the rigours of asylum life that they died soon after retiring.
Significantly, the attendants felt that they too were 'confined' in the
asylum, and regarded their work as dangerous and trying, with few
compensations.

Unrest was rife in the 1890s in the London county asylums and in
Ireland, where unsuccessful attempts were made to establish trade
unions. At Storthes Hall, the authorities were concerned enough
expressly to forbid trade unionism among their staff. Rule 58 ran:

any discussion or other proceeding with a view to, or in the nature
of a combination among Nurses or Servants, for any object
connected with their duties or position in the Asylum, unless with
the cognizance and sanction of the Medical Superintendent is
strictly prohibited; and every Nurse or Servant joining therein, will
be liable to dismissal . . .[55]

A widening gulf was appearing between the men and women who
possessed the greatest responsibility for patient care and those in formal
charge of the institution. At a time when wages were under £50 a year,
it was not uncommon for a medical superintendent of a large asylum to
receive £800 a year and, in addition, a fine house and the pick of the
farm's produce. Staff were not always slow to detect the hypocrisy of
authorities who publicly expressed high ideals, but left staff to struggle
on with minimal resources. The managers of asylums sponsored the
Asylum Workers' Association (AWA), an organisation which portrayed,
in the *Asylum News*, an idealised image of asylum life, and encouraged
staff to believe they had an identity of interest with their superiors. The

AWA was not a democratic organisation. Its affairs were dominated by medical superintendents. One of the few nurses influential in its affairs was Honnor Morton, a general trained nurse and pupil of Miss Lückes.[56] Morton sought to implant notions of professionalism from the outside, and placed mental nursing high in the hierarchy of nursing occupations:

> Surely if it be well to be a home nurse, and capable of taking care of one's relations, it is better to be a hospital nurse, and equal to attending to the stranger who is physically ill; but it is best to be an asylum nurse and minister to the mind diseased.[57]

The rank-and-file staff largely rejected these views, as they rejected, in the end, the AWA. They often viewed such idealised images of asylum employment as the fantasies of those who were typically cosseted from the stresses and strains of daily life in the wards. Inherent in this response was a negative evaluation of their work and an instrumental (i.e. economic) orientation that is often disturbingly frank. An anonymous attendant poet, writing in the *National Asylum Workers' Union Magazine* was moved to ask in verse 'why men with wealth and power delight to be unjust', saying that workers' 'souls are shrivelled and destroyed in the unceasing strife/To gain the few necessities to save their bodies life'. The poet continued:

> It is the wretched victims of their poison in life's cup,
> Who in increasing numbers fill these vast Asylums up;
> And with this human wreckage we are herded all day long.
> For all the hours heav'n sends us must we mix with this and throng.
> Repulsive work we have to do, and bear obscene abuse,
> And undergo a mental strain from which there is no truce;
> Our tempers through the live long day are tried full a time;
> But if we make the slightest slip 'tis counted as a crime.
> Small are our wages, and our food oft times unfit to eat;
> While soul-degrading tyranny our mis'ry doth complete.

The author then castigated what seemed the self-evident hypocrisy of their 'masters' who

> ... Christian virtues show in caring for the weak;
> But of the money that it costs for mercy's sake don't speak.
> They get terrific brain-storms when they think of the expense,
> In which their Christian virtues fly a very long way hence.

They say 'The sorrows of these creatures almost make us weep,
And we must ease their sufferings, but we must do it cheap:
So down we'll keep the wages bill by all means in our power,
There's plenty glad to get a job at nothing much an hour.[58]

It was this kind of perspective on their work which led asylum
attendants to regard their work as a form of wage labour, and which
gave rise to a trade union consciousness. An 'official' response to this
growing movement from 1910 was expressed by an article in *The
Hospital* in 1913. Expressing its horror against attempts to represent
'the interests of the superior officers, as opposed to that of the rank
and file', its author ended with an appeal to asylum workers:

to remember that theirs is a 'high calling' and that the tending and
nursing of the insane, exacting as it does, the best qualities of heart
and head, hardly falls under the same category as the daily job of the
labourer or even the mechanic.

These remarks caused some hilarity in union circles. The intangible
rewards of professionalism were not seen as an adequate compensation
for low wages, poor conditions and harsh discipline. One male
correspondent to the union magazine expressed the following
sentiment:

Why should you grumble because a tradesman works 50 hours a week
and you 80 or 90 or more? Have you not your *dignity*? Cling to that
precious position; feed the wife and children with it when pay-day is
approaching; when the coalman comes with his bill, try paying him
with a 'dignified' look. If the 'Super' has you up for some little
offence, ask him how he dares meddle with one engaged in a
'dignified profession'. Grievances vanish and sorrows fade before the
wonderful zephyr of dignity.[59]

It seems that male workers were much more likely to reject
professional ideology: they certainly joined the union in greater
numbers in the early days. Women nurses were more likely to adhere to
professional and vocational values. The *NAWU Magazine*, in fact,
contemptuously described the Asylum Workers' Association as the
'Asylum *Womens'* Association'. In part this reflected the higher class
background of some nurses and their background in general nursing.
Yet, at the margins, the sex of the nurse was probably significant in

determining occupational attitudes, but not because of any inherent differences. Perhaps the culturally sanctioned expectation of self-sacrifice among women was more influential among female nurses, while men seemed to have scorned it.

The most striking difference between the sexes, however, was that women were much less likely to join the union or the AWA. The male attendants, through the letter columns of the *NA WU Magazine*, sometimes complained that women would not join the union because they were not prepared to stand up to authority. But too much weight can be given to such arguments. There were more material differences in the situation of men's and women's employment in the asylum. Men were much more likely to stay once they had joined the service. They thus formed a stable recruitment base for the union. On the female side, turnover of staff was very high, in some cases 30 per cent a year. Mental nursing, as we have seen, failed to attract more than a small group of career-orientated women to its ranks. For the vast majority who entered it during this period, asylum nursing did not form a permanent or even semi-permanent career. Such circumstances create stony ground for any kind of occupational association; workers are difficult to recruit in the first place, and in any case may soon leave the service. These problems are, of course, not unknown to modern-day trade unionists in the health service.

Despite wishful thinking in high places that asylum nursing could mirror general nursing in achieving public honour and dignity, work in asylums was considered largely to be a degrading occupation, not just by nurses but by the world at large. This general view has not disappeared. Mental nursing is still not a glamorous occupation; how many soap operas and romantic love stories are set in mental hospitals?

If asylum work was generally regarded as degrading, it was only to be expected that most staff would also see it in such terms. A society which shunned, excluded and confined the mentally disturbed had no right to expect very different attitudes from those it recruited, at low wages and poor conditions, to look after them. Asylum work was 'dirty' work which, as Everett Hughes has emphasised, is not only or mainly physically dirty, but also personally degrading to those who perform it, because 'it in some way goes counter to the more heroic of our moral conceptions'.[60] Much of general nursing was physically dirty and potentially degrading. But nursing reform partially transformed nursing tasks – or rather, transformed those performing them into dignified and heroic 'angels'. Those who tended the mentally disturbed, however, have never been publicly regarded as heroic, even though they often risked their health and sometimes their lives on behalf of a society which largely took their efforts for granted. Fine-sounding phrases could do little to remedy that neglect. What was required, and what emerged, was a vigorous social movement among rank-and-file staff, determined to win fair treatment and rewards through the only effective means open to them: trade union organisation and activity.

Notes

1. I am grateful to the Confederation of Health Service Employees for providing the funds which made this research possible. In this chapter I deal only with nursing in public asylums. The continuing programme of research will be widened to include the nursing of the mentally disturbed in workhouses and private asylums. The development of mental handicap nursing will also be traced.

2. A. Walk, 'The History of Mental Nursing', *Journal of Mental Science* (1961), pp. 1–17.

3. A. Gouldner, *The Coming Crisis of Western Sociology* (Heinemann, London, 1970), Ch. 13.

4. B. Abel-Smith, *A History of the Nursing Profession* (Heinemann, London, 1960).

5. M. Foucault, *Madness and Civilisation: A History of Insanity in the Age of Reason* (Tavistock, London, 1961), p. ix.

6. Ibid.

7. Quoted by Foucault, ibid.

8. M. Fears, 'Therapeutic Optimism and the Treatment of the Insane', in R. Dingwall *et al.* (eds), *Health Care and Health Knowledge* (Croom Helm, London, 1977), pp. 66–81.

9. From S. Tuke, *Description of the Retreat* (1813), reprinted in C. Goshen, *A Documentary History of Psychiatry* (Vision Press, London, 1967).

10. W. Battie, *A Treatise on Madness* (1757), reprinted in part in Goshen, *Documentary History*.

11. Ibid.

12. Tuke, *Description of the Retreat*.

13. J. Conolly, *The Construction and Government of Lunatic Asylums and Hospitals for the Insane* (1847), reprinted Dawson of Pall Mall (London, 1968), p. 83.

14. Foucault, *Madness and Civilisation*, pp. 251–2.

15. *Handbook for Attendants on the Insane*, 5th edn (Balliere, Tindall and Cox, London, 1908), p. 373.

16. Ibid., p. 323.

17. Ibid., p. 363.

18. Ibid., p. 315.

19. A. Scull, *Museums of Madness: The Social Organisation of Insanity in 19th Century England* (Allen Lane, London, 1979), p. 219.

20. G. Pearson, *The Deviant Imagination* (Macmillan, London, 1977), p. 164.

21. Ibid., p. 161.

22. *Report of the Medical Superintendent, Prestwich County Asylum* (February 1875), Lancashire Records Office.

23. *Regulations and Orders for the Government of the Wiltshire County Asylum, Devizes* (1882).

24. *County of London Asylums Committee: Manual of Duties* (1906).

25. R. Hunter, 'The Rise and Fall of Mental Nursing', in *In the Mental Hospital: Articles Reprinted from the Lancet* (*The Lancet*, London, 1955), pp. 54–9.

26. T. A. Critchley, *A History of Police in England and Wales* (Constable, London, 1978), p. 38.

27. Department of Employment, *British Labour Statistics* (HMSO, London, 1971), p. 38.

28. Ibid., p. 28; note that the figures are for rates, not earnings, which may have been even higher.

29. J. Rowe, *Wages in Theory and Practice* (George Routledge, London, 1928), p. 35; rates, not earnings.

30. Abel-Smith, *Nursing Profession*, p. 280.

31. Cited by John Burnett, in *Useful Toil* (Allen Lane, London, 1971), p. 161.

32. J. Kuczynski, *A Short History of Labour Conditions Under Industrial Capitalism in Great Britain and the Empire 1750–1944* (Frederick Muller, London, 1972), p. 92.

33. Conolly, *Construction and Government of Lunatic Asylums*, p. 86.

34. See E. Santos and E. Stainbrook, 'A History of Psychiatric Nursing in the 19th Century, I–II', *Journal of the History of Medicine and Allied Sciences*, IV (1949), pp. 48–73.

35. *Select Committee on Asylum Officers (Employment, Pensions and Superannuation) Bill, 1911*, minutes of evidence.

36. 'The Future of the Asylum Service', *Medical Press and Circular*, 21 March 1900.

37. Ibid., 28 March 1900.

38. F. Adams, 'From Association to Union: Professional Organisation of Asylum Attendants 1869–1919', *British Journal of Sociology*, 20 (1969), pp. 11–26.

39. Quoted by K. Jones, *Lunacy, Law and Conscience, 1744–1855* (Routledge and Kegan Paul, London, 1955), p. 159.

40. H. Burdett, *Hospitals and Asylums of the World*, vol. 1 (J. and A. Churchill, London), p. 630.

41. Conolly, *Construction and Government of Lunatic Asylums*, p. 86.

42. Quoted by Burdett, *Hospitals and Asylums*, p. 632.

43. *Asylum News* (1900), pp. 42–3.

44. Ibid. (1918), p. 35.

45. Edith Morley (ed.), *Women Workers in Seven Professions* (George Routledge, London, 1914), p. 201. The chapter on nursing was written by Miss E. M. Musson.

46. A. Gouldner, *Patterns of Industrial Bureaucracy* (Routledge and Kegan Paul, London, 1955).

47. *Regulations and Orders for the Management and Conduct of those Engaged in the Service of the Middlesex County Asylum, Napsbury* (1905).

48. Metropolitan Asylums Board, *Imbecile Asylums: Staff Regulations* (1901).

49. Source: Lancashire Records Office, Preston.

50. Scull, *Museums of Madness*, Ch. 5.

51. T. Scheff, 'Control Over Policy by Attendants in a Mental Hospital', *Journal of Health and Human Behaviour*, 2 (1961), pp. 93–105.

52. M. Lomax, *The Experience of an Asylum Doctor* (George Allen and Unwin, London, 1921), p. 98.

53. Cited in ibid.

54. C. Andrews, *The Dark Awakening: A History of St. Andrews Hospital, Bodmin* (The Hospital, Bodmin, 1978), p. 93.

55. Storthes Hall Asylum, Kirkburton, near Huddersfield, *Regulations and Orders of the Committee of Visitors for the Management and Conduct of the Asylum* (1904).

56. Miss Lückes was matron of the London Hospital for many years and a leading figure in the late-nineteenth-century nursing world.

57. *Asylum News*, May 1900.

58. *National Asylum Workers' Union Magazine*, February 1912.

59. *NAWU Magazine*, May 1912.

60. Everett Hughes, *Men and Their Work* (New York Free Press, 1958), p. 50.

7 'THE HISTORY OF THE PRESENT' — CONTRADICTION AND STRUGGLE IN NURSING

Paul Bellaby and Patrick Oribabor

At first sight, this chapter seems not to belong in a history volume at all. For, after some critical comments on the writing of history, there is an analysis of questionnaire data concerning present-day membership of professional associations and trade unions which proceeds much in the manner of survey sociology. But then the direction changes; Bellaby and Oribabor reveal their dissatisfaction with this approach and look to history to illuminate the patterns they have found. They conduct what they call a 'reciprocal' study of past and present. They take the 1930s, a period when union solidarity was strong, and scrutinise it in detail. They examine the nature and control of nursing work and the broader economic context and relate these two to each other and to the struggles and strategies in trade unions and professional associations at the time. They then try to apply their analysis to the present day, arguing that current issues have a different content but can be understood via the same style of analysis.

Some readers will wish for more material on the 1970s. Others will want to ask whether the analysis stresses class divisions at the expense of sexual ones. Still others — like myself — who have stressed direct continuities in nursing history will need to think again. Whatever one's final judgements, these authors certainly show that new interpretations can be drawn from old material — provided the questions one starts with are different.

—————Ed.

(Why study the past?) Simply because I am interested in the past? No, if one means by that writing a history of the past in terms of the present. Yes, if one means writing the *history of the present*.

M. Foucault[1]

Much can be learned about the problems of writing a history of nursing by considering what may at first appear an unlikely parallel. It concerns the relation between the Tiv of Nigeria and their colonial rulers. When disputes were brought to the district courts, the Tiv evoked their genealogies in support of their cases. These were transmitted from generation to generation by word of mouth. However, before the first war, colonial officials had written down and collated the family trees mentioned in court cases. Forty years later, the same records were used by the courts themselves to adjudicate competing claims. By this time, the Tiv maintained that the records were inaccurate.

If Tiv dissatisfaction with the court records is put in context, it can be seen that the genealogies they had evoked forty years previously no longer corresponded to the constitution of Tiv society. Some lines mentioned in the old family trees were no longer extant, while new lines had appeared and the pecking order among lineages had altered. Presumably, if left to themselves, the Tiv would have modified their genealogies, so as to legitimate the present order of their society: not necessarily in the manner of the ruling class in Orwell's *1984*, but simply because old memories fade. By writing down the genealogies of forty years previously, the colonial officials had ossified what would otherwise be a living tradition.[2]

Like the family trees of the Tiv, histories of nursing often constitute a search for origins, and they sometimes have an apologetic or congratulatory tone. This invites the (unconscious) intrusion of present interests into the reconstruction of the past, for this kind of scholarship pulls one strand from the tangle of present society and follows it back, while, in starting the written account from the origin of that strand, implying that history has moved continuously to the point at which the author believes we now stand. For example, many of the more popular accounts focus on the development of training, on state registration and on the extent of employment of trained nurses.[3] This focus corresponds to one interest, but only one, in the current struggles of nursing as an occupation – the claim to professional standing. It is possible to take out other strands. Thus White fixes her attention on the neglected majority of British nurses who, prior to 1930, were employed under the poor law and, after that date, by local authorities.[4] The 'present interest' in this theme is the legacy it is presumed to have left to community nursing and to the hospital nursing of the chronic sick, especially the aged. Nursing within the asylums might form another strand.[5] Finally, we might take trade unionism rather than professionalism as the topical interest and trace its origins and developments.[6]

Such an alternation of focus can make for lively debate among historians and practitioners alike. However, the reader can be forgiven for seeing the separate histories as competing claims as to what the origins of nursing were or, even, what nursing is. It tends to pass unnoticed that in fact there are several strands in both current and past nursing; that nursing is and has been divided in various ways, rather than unified; and that groups of nurses have from time to time found themselves in contradictory situations, left to agonise as to what tactics they should adopt. It is this contradictory texture of the states of nursing, past and present, that is the focus of our paper.

The study of the past has a particular significance for 'historical materialism',[7] the method which guides this paper. It helps reveal the specific nature of the present. Prevailing ideas (ideology) make the arrangements in which we live appear natural and immutable. By focusing on the discontinuities between past and present, we can set ourselves outside that ideology. More pertinently, by asking what had to change to bring about the state in which we now live (or practice as nurses), it reveals the underlying mechanisms of present-day society: the present as history, in the words of Lukács.[8]

However, the very question — 'what had to change to bring about the present?' — is refined by growing knowledge of the present itself. The greater our knowledge of the present, the more relevant can be our inquiries into the past. There is thus a reciprocal relation between historical and current studies, a relation that can be found in many Marxist classics, but is perhaps less widely pursued than it should be.[9] With this in mind, we begin the substantive analysis in this paper in an unorthodox way, by laying out what, as it were innocent of history, we have culled about the present struggles of nursing from a social survey. We are then drawn to historical analysis to interpret the survey itself.

The Present: as if apart from History

The social survey that we shall briefly consider here was concerned with membership of unions and professional associations among nurses. It was carried out by one of the authors during 1977/78. It was centred on nurses working in five wards — each representing a different specialism — within one small Area Health Authority (AHA). Three of the specialisms — general medicine, pre- and post-operative surgery, and an intensive therapy unit (ITU) — were situated in the 'infirmary', our pseudonym for the former voluntary hospital in the AHA. The other two — acute psychiatry and acute/chronic geriatrics — were on a separate site, a bus ride from the infirmary, but still in the city that was the core of the AHA: this site was being developed as a district general hospital complex, but the original buildings had been the former poor law/municipal hospital before nationalisation. We have called this site 'city'. Seventy-seven clinical nurses were interviewed in the survey, and they were also observed at work; line management and the Rcn and union stewards or representatives were also interviewed.

The AHA is here known as 'Westmid'.[10]

Our analysis of the survey proceeds on three levels. On one level we seek to establish the regularity (or rules-followed) in the reasons nurses gave for joining a union or the Royal College of Nursing (Rcn). This is only one possible cause of the pattern of membership. At a second level, because the mere presence of organisation in a work-setting increases the likelihood of unionisation, we must consider the local activities of unions and professional associations and their impact on potential members. Finally, there is a range of factors concerned with the employment of nurses — pay, the organisation of work, the control system and so on — which the survey gives an opportunity to examine. The survey allows us only to infer possible causes, especially of the remoter kind. This is partly because of its small scope and not necessarily representative nature, but largely because, like all surveys, it shows a cross-section at one point in time. Of course, when survey specialists speak of 'explaining' the variation, say, in union/Rcn membership, they imply that certain co-variations (as between member-ship and reasons for joining) are, on common-sense or theoretical grounds, to be treated as if cause and effect. To move from what is really inference to more grounded knowledge calls for longitudinal (or over-time) studies. Thus survey analysis can only pave the way to 'historical' work.

The Rcn, the Trade Unions and their Membership in Westmid

Of the 77 clinical nurses in the survey, all but seven were members of either the Rcn or a trade union. Given that six in every seven of these nurses was a woman and, in general, women are less likely to join organisations of this kind than men, this is a striking degree of 'completeness', or level of membership among potential members.

A further feature of membership in Westmid is that no fewer than four organisations were represented. All are registered as trade unions, though in the case of the Rcn registration dates only from June 1977. It is, however, convenient to group the others as 'trade unions', and thus imply a contrast with the Rcn, because in many ways the Rcn is not a typical trade union in the character of its policies and organisation, while the others, by and large, are so.[11] The other three are affiliated to the TUC, while the Rcn has merely considered affiliation (and recently rejected it). Two of them, the National Association of Local and Government Officers (NALGO) and the National Union of Public Employees (NUPE), recruit across the public services, and, though NALGO is predominantly white collar and NUPE predominantly manual, NUPE has a substantial minority of white-collar members. The third union, the Confederation of Health Service Employees (COHSE), as the name implies, views itself as the industrial union of the NHS. The Rcn, however, represents only nurses and restricts membership to those trained or in training (this has the effect of excluding the untrained nursing auxiliaries). Correspondingly, the Rcn considers the advance of standards of performance and conduct, of formal education and of research in nursing, to be some of its central functions. None of the unions has similar commitments. Another way in which the Rcn differs from the trade unions is that the leadership deplores 'militancy' — in particular, use of the strike — a position linked in this context with emphasis on the responsibility of nurses, as professionals, to their patients. Excluding the auxiliaries, of the 62 clinical nurses in the Westmid sample who were eligible for Rcn membership, only ten actually belonged. In principle nurses might combine Rcn with union membership, but none did so. The strongest trade unions among the nurses here were NALGO (29 members) and NUPE (22), while COHSE had one member fewer than the Rcn (nine). The small membership of COHSE is no less remarkable than the small membership of the Rcn, for, just as the latter claims to be the nurses' own association, so COHSE claims to represent NHS workers as a whole.

As a matter of fact, the distinction between the Rcn and the trade unions will be overdrawn if we confine attention to its ideology of 'professionalism'. The Rcn also acts as a trade union. From the outset of the NHS in 1948, it has been extremely well represented on the Whitley Council, a body set up to negotiate the salaries and terms of employment of nurses. Currently the Rcn commands eight of the 18 seats on the Nurses' and Midwives' Functional Council (NUPE and COHSE have four each, and NALGO two). Of late it has developed a 'steward' structure, intended to compete with those of trade unions, and the leadership has been much exercised over the ethics of 'militancy' and whether the Rcn should affiliate to the TUC.

Why Join the Rcn/a Union?

Nurses' own Reasons.   We can begin to answer the two questions of why membership was so complete and yet so scattered among different organisations by turning to the reasons that nurses gave for joining. On the whole, the few Rcn members gave one set of reasons and the trade union members gave another set. This difference seems to flow from the ways in which the two types of organisation are constituted — their 'character' — except that the 'trade union' side of the Rcn seems to make little impression on its rank and file.

All the Rcn members said that belonging to the College expressed solidarity with other nurses, that the Rcn was the champion of nursing standards. Eight of the ten gave 'education' as a further reason for joining. Eight also said that they would not join a strike under any circumstances, as, interestingly enough, did all seven nurses who belonged to no organisation.

Union members for the most part accepted the possibility of strike action. But a substantial minority (19 of the 60) were against it whatever the circumstances, and 30 of the 41 who said they would join a strike implied that they would do so with reluctance and only as a last resort, in view of the effect on patients. Furthermore, only 17 gave solidarity with other health workers as a reason for joining their union. As will be apparent, nurses' attraction to unions was expressed largely in 'instrumental' terms, though pay was by no means the only factor, local representation being at least equal to it.

The different images of the Rcn and the unions entertained by their members were by and large shared by other nurses too. All the nurses who belonged to no organisation, and fully half of the union members, acknowledged that the Rcn was the sole defender of nursing standards. Conversely, few gave the Rcn credit for its role in trade union areas. No one thought the Rcn *more* effective here than trade unions; only four felt it might be *as* effective, either in pay issues or in handling local disputes, while 28 felt it had as great a part to play in improving work conditions as had the unions, presumably because of an implied link between these conditions and 'nursing standards'.

Local Organisation as a Cause of Recruitment.   Once one starts to look beyond the reasons nurses gave for their own membership, the immediate question must be whether the vigour and efficiency of the recruitment drives of local organisations, or in addition the 'snowball' effect' on nurses in a particular ward or hospital once their peers have begun to join, might account for the completeness and scatter of membership.

The Rcn's record of recruitment at Westmid in recent years was poor. Only two of the nurses in the sample had joined in the last four years. Conversely, no fewer than 48 of the 60 union members had joined in this period: clearly there had been a large and rapid increase in union membership. There is evidence that this does reflect the efficiency of local officers. For instance, seven of the ten Rcn members said that since joining they had seen the Rcn steward (or her equivalent) rarely or never. By contrast, 19 of the 31 who belonged either to NUPE or COHSE claimed that they saw their local officers 'regularly'; and 14 of the 29 NALGO members that they saw theirs 'occasionally'.

The 'snowball effect' may well have operated among learners, all of whom joined NALGO, though they seem to have taken little interest in union affairs after joining. Elsewhere, it was confined to the two specialisms at 'city' hospital, psychiatry and geriatrics, if what counts as evidence of this is the extent to which a single organisation monopolised membership. Seven of the eight psychiatric nurses and 13 of the 22 geriatric nurses belonged to a single union (COHSE and NUPE respectively); and five of the nurses on geriatrics who did not belong to NUPE were learners undergoing a temporary placement there. Unlike most learners, and also most of the nurses in the other specialisms, all of them at the infirmary, those in psychiatry and geriatrics were relatively committed to their union. They were more likely to attend meetings, keep up with the journal and see their representatives.

The 'snowball effect' may be interpreted in one of two ways: either as evidence of a somewhat superficial commitment to membership, or else as evidence of a movement that gathers force in individual consciousness and collectively as members join. Such as the evidence is, it would appear that, while learners probably fell into the first category, a high proportion of recruits in psychiatry and geriatrics fell into the latter. In both psychiatry and geriatrics, nurses wore union badges and freely discussed union affairs. By contrast, infirmary nurses were inhibited about displaying their affiliation because they sensed the disapproval of superiors. It is they, presumably, who were the more 'instrumental' and individuated in their motives for joining.

It would appear, then, that local organisation and informal pressure were factors in the successful recruitment policies of trade unions. However, this can hardly be a sufficient explanation of the rapid rise of union membership, if only because the Rcn could in principle have recruited all but the 15 auxiliaries who were not eligible to join, and indeed had made in the critical period some national efforts to change local structures. The clue to the puzzle must lie in the unfavourable view the nurses took of the Rcn's capacity to act as a trade union. Putting it another way, we have to ask what promoted a demand on the part of nurses for union tactics, for something that the Rcn could not give them. The customary cross-sectional method of the survey — measuring attitudes, comparing group with group — can provide some insights into possible causes here, though a definitive answer must rest on historical research.

Might Pay have been a Decisive Issue?   Another way of interpreting the fact that the unions recruited four-fifths of their members either in 1974 or subsequently is to lay stress on the coincidence of this with a period of inflation that left nurses in a position where their standard of living may have been declining and certainly where 'differentials' with other groups were being squeezed. In particular, 1974 was the year of a dispute with government over nurses' pay.[12] In the sample as a whole, 51 (out of 77) considered their pay poor or very poor. This included 44 of the 60 union members, but only seven of the 17 who either belonged to the Rcn or to no organisation. Furthermore, when asked what they felt unions/the Rcn should be doing for nursing, and given the opportunity to say anything, without prompting, 37 of the unionists, but only four of the Rcn members and non-members, said the defence of pay was important.

On theoretical grounds, one should hesitate to let pay bear the main burden of explanation here. First, in general pay is often a rallying cry for a wide range of grievances, the more so as it can be broached without impugning managers one must work with daily and allows bargaining in quantities rather than feelings.[13] Secondly, nursing has several peculiarities which make one call for an account of how pay might become an issue at all. It is predominantly women's work. Further, there is a strong sense among nurses that theirs is a calling, and the almost universal public admiration for nurses is based on their reputation for selfless devotion to their patients. Admittedly, this public support has proved an asset in nurses' struggles for pay that matches their responsibilities and against exploitation of their good nature. But it remains a block on seeking improvements in pay in the first place. Thus we must explore other factors that might explain the emergence of pay at a particular time as a rallying cry.

Is Management Control a Factor?   Dissatisfaction with management was widespread (56 mentioned it spontaneously); usually this reflected a sense that management was remote and impersonal. Indeed, all nurses but two said they felt powerless to influence what happened to them in the hospital. Specifically, they had in mind a policy, pursued with somewhat varied rigour from ward to ward, of making nurses sign for the treatment they gave. In a context in which (in their eyes) patients and their relatives were encouraged to make complaints to management, close accountability laid individuals open to invidious discipline. In such a situation we would expect nurses to look to vigorous union officials to act as intermediaries with management.

By 'management', it transpired, clinical nurses understood not only the hospital administrators properly so-called, but also nurses of nursing officer grade and above. It is striking that among the latter, the Rcn was stronger than for any other level of nursing at Westmid. Only one nursing officer (and above) belonged to no organisation; of the other 16, no fewer than twelve belonged to the Rcn; the remainder were NALGO members. It seems plausible that the Rcn was identified with 'management' and, since clinical nurses felt their interests to be different from those of management, they joined other organisations when their interests were threatened.

Is the Organisation of Work a Factor? Nurses were observed at work and also asked about their work relations with supervisors. We shall not attempt a detailed analysis of the survey data here; this has been presented elsewhere.[14] What is important for our present analysis is the relationship between nurses' experiences of work and their membership of organisations.

In all specialisms there was a finely spaced hierarchy of status and control among nurses, but there were variations in the pattern of work from specialism to specialism. Psychiatry and geriatrics were distinct from the others. Nurses there were 'care' oriented and performed a relatively wide and diffuse range of tasks. They enjoyed a sphere of control over the patient, independent of medicine. Their counterparts in medicine, surgery and the ITU were 'cure' oriented and performed a definite and quite narrow range of tasks. Their work was routinised and under the more direct control of medicine. They developed through their work less of a sense of corporate identity than did nurses in psychiatry and geriatrics.

The pattern of Rcn/union membership reflected these features of the organisation of work. In the ITU, surgical and medical nurses (all on the infirmary site) belonged to different unions or the Rcn depending on the grade. For example, six of the eight sisters belonged to the Rcn while six of the seven auxiliaries who belonged to organisations were scattered among all three of the unions. In psychiatry and geriatrics (the specialisms in the city site) sisters and auxiliaries belonged by and large to the same organisation. But for one sister, all these nurses belonged either to COHSE (if in psychiatry) or NUPE (if in geriatrics).

A possible way of carrying forward the difference we find here is to ask two questions of historical research. The first is whether what we have discovered at Westmid is a long-standing distinction between the social organisation of work in these two groups of specialisms that may,

in its turn, account for different responses to the factors that have
brought the spurt of union membership. The second is whether the
specialisms indicate, on a yet longer time-scale, uneven development in
nursing as a whole in one direction or the other — towards greater
specificity or greater diffuseness, towards greater independence of
medicine or more medical control.

However, the distinction between specialisms, and also the
difference between grades, affects which organisation people join, not
whether they join *an* organisation. Thus, of the possible causes we have
considered, some change in management and the emergence of pay as
an issue seem the most likely to account for the growth of unionism
per se.

History of the Present

The analysis of the survey points to possible lines of historical inquiry.
Of itself, it gives little information about the processes by which nurses
were mobilised in unions and the Rcn, or of the unfolding of their
struggles. Further, though we can infer possible causes of unionisation
from the survey, we cannot demonstrate that these 'causes' actually led
to that outcome. Nor are we in a position to determine how far the
present situation is unique and of recent origin rather than similar to
situations in the past and a development from the past. The one likely
source of parallels to the present situation in nursing is the emergence
of unionism in the 1930s.

Unfortunately, the sources for Westmid's history are too fragmentary
to allow us to reconstruct local events in the 1930s. We can only trace
the broad national picture at that time. On the other hand, the pattern
that we have found in Westmid at present seems in most respects quite
typical of the country as a whole.[15] Accordingly, while our account of
the 1930s is only national in scope, that of the present at Westmid can
be treated as a sample of the present national situation.

Contradictions in the Past Struggles of Nurses

Most people would concede that at present nursing is internally
divided about professionalism and unionism, and, even among unionists,
about which union to join. But it has been quite common to view the
past as a period of unity under a single leadership — at least after the
1919 Registration Act. From that point the 'profession' of nursing is
supposed to have come to power.

Professionalism v. Unionism.   The present division among nurses is
not new. The late 1930s were marked by a growth of union membership. This is difficult to quantify, but it was sufficient to be seen as a
threat by the leadership of professional associations and to make
unions representing nurses (along with other health workers) a
persuasive voice in the Trade Union Congress.

The public contest between professional associations and trade
unions was joined over a bill presented to Parliament on the initiative
of unions organising in the health services in April 1937. It reinvigorated
a proposal made by the labour movement several times since the First
World War for a fixed working week for all health workers (excepting
doctors). The Rcn urged MPs to oppose the bill. In its riposte, the TUC
attacked the Rcn for denying membership to male nurses, student
nurses and nurses on the GNC supplementary registers (all of which
was true), implying that it represented the voluntary hospitals and, out
of snobbery, excluded the nurses who were preponderant in local
authority hospitals (former poor law infirmaries and county asylums).
On closer inspection it is clear that the Rcn opposed the bill because it
felt regulation of hours was incompatible with being professional and in
broader terms, as the *Nursing Times* put it, on the issue of whether
nurses should 'throw in their lot with other workers who chance to be
employed at the same institution or by the same employer'.[16]

This contradiction between professional associations representing
nurses (of which the Rcn was by then the chief) and trade unions
representing a mixed group of health workers was overlaid by another.
The hospitals were trying to recruit far more nurses than the training
schools could then produce. Already (by 1937) there were almost as
many untrained people doing basic nursing in hospitals as there were
nurses on the general register currently employed in the hospitals. The
registered nurses were to be found disproportionately in the hospitals,
which were largely voluntary as indeed were the training schools
approved by the GNC. Untrained people were employed chiefly in the
large infirmaries inherited by the local authorities from the poor law in
the 1930s, in the TB sanitoria and in the asylums. These institutions
were expanding in the 1930s. They made up as best they could for the
stigma that was attached to work with the mentally ill and chronically
ill, by offering wages at a premium above those of voluntary hospitals.
Even so they had difficulty both in recruiting trained nurses and in
enrolling students and retaining them. Less stringent requirements for
registration than those laid down by the GNC and upheld by the
professional associations would clearly be to their advantage.

Despite a substantial difference in goals and tactics, unions and professional associations alike responded to this market situation. Trained nurses lacked a monopoly over the labour used in the hospital to nurse the sick. If they had had such a monopoly they would have been able to force up their price (however they wanted it to be paid — in status and control if not in money). Lacking it, they had two alternatives when faced with demand that exceeded their capacity to supply. The first was to permit further dilution of their labour, hoping to push up the price for trained nursing as the price of untrained labour rose. This was the explicit tactic of the unions. They tried to lift the wages of the lowest paid and, in so far as they were concerned with higher grades, to pass this advantage on by repairing 'differentials'. The second tactic was adopted by the Rcn and the other professional associations, namely to try and conserve the degree of control that trained nurses already had over entry into the profession. Now this control was precarious, both externally, in relation to the authorities and medicine, and internally, in relation to rank-and-file nurses. As we shall see, focus on conserving control led the professional associations into what appears at first sight anything but market behaviour, such as trying to keep down the wages of student nurses. Nevertheless, the contradictory market position was as much the basis of their tactics as it was of those of the unions.

The contest involving the Rcn and the unions in the late 1930s had an outcome more favourable to the Rcn than to the unions. The main reason was that the Rcn shifted its ground. Whereas the Rcn and the Matrons' Association had previously insisted on a single portal of entry to nursing, they now conceded the possibility of a second — the shorter training of the 'assistant nurses'.[17] Though this particular grade proved of limited importance, the concession of principle opened up the possibility of accommodating the influx of non-nurses who nevertheless nursed, within a hierarchic division of labour headed by SRNs — the 'grade system'. It also allowed the professional associations to go some way towards meeting the demand of hospital authorities for more nurses, while appearing to preserve its insistence on standards. The Rcn was subsequently prominent on wartime committees and was able to gain more favourable representation than the unions on the Whitley Council for nursing.

Within the period from the first war to the founding of the NHS, professional associations and unions pursued their differing policies within the space opened by the hospitals' buoyant demand for nursing labour. However, the contradictory situation they confronted not only sustained the contrary policies of unionism and professionalism – it also affected the strategies of each.

Contradictions within Professionalism. Since the claim to be professional is also a claim to high social standing, it is to be expected that the term will be used in varied ways in different instances. Clearly it is of no concern to the sociologist to pass judgement for or against such claims. Indeed, if the term is to be used at all in sociology, it must have an exact meaning. Among the most useful attempts to construct a typology in which professionalism can have a definite place is that of Johnson.[18] His approach is also consistent with historical materialism. He placed professionalism within the relation between the producer of a service or goods and the consumer. The uncertainties in that relation, such as, in the case of health care, the needs of the patient and the appropriate treatment, may be variously controlled: by producer, by consumer or by third party. Plainly, professionalism takes the form of the producer's control (defining the consumer's needs and how they should be treated) where the producer acts as one of a recognised group of 'colleagues'. The establishment of a profession depends upon external factors[19] – breaking loose from the patronage of consumers, gaining a monopoly over a sphere of practice and establishing the means to defend it (usually in law), freedom from intervention by third parties – and internal factors – means of socialising and disciplining members.

Even before the Registration Act of 1919, the Nightingale reform had established, chiefly in the voluntary hospital, an impressive measure of internal control. Training resembled that of a novitiate in a monastic order; the matron controlled every aspect of the nurse's work and leisure, both of which were conducted within the hospital boundaries. However, so complete was the subordination of the individual nurse to the nursing structure that was symbolised by the matron that it cannot be said that individually nurses exerted any control over patients. Nursing was a well-disciplined corps but not a 'group' of colleagues. Did nursing really achieve external autonomy and control? For many historians (including Abel-Smith) there seem to be parallels between the 1919 Act and the 1858 Act which set up the medical register. When this is examined within the theoretical framework we have set up, the similarities disappear and the level of autonomy and control in nursing has to be questioned.

First, as is already apparent from our discussion to date of the unionism of those excluded from the general register, registration did not unify nursing. The College did not succeed in organising nursing as a whole under the leadership of those who were trained. The diversity of circumstances of employment for voluntary hospital and public sector nurses underlay this contradiction between the precept of 'unity' and the practice of diversity.

Secondly, throughout the inter-war period, there was a struggle for leadership of registered nurses themselves. This turned on whether nursing should, rather than acting as a corps of assistants to doctors, strike out as a distinctively female profession, working alongside but not subordinate to medicine, and distinguished by a higher standard of training than currently provided. Arguably, Mrs Fenwick and her followers, who took this view, acknowledged more sharply than their successful competitors (the College of Nursing principally) the contradictory nature of claiming professional standing when acting within a framework established by another profession.[20] With some important variation (which we shall consider below), doctors mediated in the relation between nurses and patients: they defined the patients' needs and the treatment appropriate to their conditions. Even if doctors had not individually ordered nurses' work, *their* ideology would have dominated the hospital.

The third contradiction was that the state, which had apparently granted a monopoly of practice to registered nurses, more or less surreptitiously ensured that no such monopoly was exercised. In her essay in this volume, Davies documents how state manipulation deprived nursing leaders of effective control over the training of nurses. An instance of this, striking enough to occasion opposition from the leadership, was the constitution and the proposals of the Wood Committee (1946–47). Though it contained two nurses, it had been set up within the ministry without consultation with the nursing organisations. It made far-reaching proposals for ending the 'novitiate' and separating training from ward work, as well as from the matron's control.[21] Broadly, there were two reasons for state interference in this and in similar instances. First, the state defended the service needs of hospitals as a priority, and these might include expanding the supply of labour for nursing, if need be by bringing in untrained nurses, let alone by shortened training; secondly, while the demand of hospitals for more staff necessarily increased spending (and even in the voluntary sector from the 1930s *public* spending), economic orthodoxy dictated restraint in 'non-productive' spending, especially where this was incurred by the state. The nursing profession was especially vulnerable to state interference, largely because it was

dependent on the state as an ally to mediate in its weak position
vis-à-vis medicine and the hospital authorities.[22]

Matrons, as local leaders, were caught in a fourth contradiction
between the interests of the nursing corps and pressures to service
hospitals, which were almost always short of funds. Hours were long
and pay was poor, especially in the voluntary sector. But this is not the
whole story. The interests of nursing, as the leaders of the 'profession'
saw it, coincided with long hours and poor pay: in the rhetoric of the
day, these protected the vocational commitments of the nurse. Of
special interest is opposition to changes either in the content of nurse
training or in the abysmal remuneration that students received for it;
this was in spite of the fact that students contributed heavily in the
supply of unskilled nursing on the ward. We suggest that the opposition
may be translated into a fear on the part of matrons that, without the
physical and mental ordeal of training, the tight internal discipline of
nursing under their control would collapse. They were right. But before
we pursue this further, we must turn from contradictions within
professionalism to contradictions within unionism in nursing.

Contradictions within Unionism.   The great majority of those
represented by 'professional associations' are, like trade unionists,
employees. The distinction between professional associations does not
necessarily correspond to labour *v.* capital or to employed producer *v.*
independent producer. Nevertheless, trade unions can be distinguished
ideologically and tactically from professional associations by the extent
to which they focus upon the employment relation and protecting their
members within it; professional associations may (like the Rcn in the
late 1930s) be responding to an underlying employment situation, but
their strategy is to achieve autonomy for the occupation they represent
— that is, independence of the employment relation or employment on
their own terms. Where the employment relation becomes of prime
importance to workers (their market position, their working conditions
or their subordination to managerial power), we can expect them to
find unionism appealing. Nevertheless, unions may be highly varied in
the constituencies they represent: perhaps a craft, where monopoly is
the bargaining power; perhaps an industry as a whole, where monopoly
can also be exercised; but most often in Britain, a conglomerate of
people in varied occupations, drawing its bargaining power and its
ability to provide services to members from its size and funds.[23]

From just before the first war to 1946, there were two main unions
to which nurses belonged which resembled the 'industrial' type. The

division between them mirrored one of several in nursing at that time: the asylum workers had one union (founded in 1910) and the workers in poor law/municipal hospitals another (founded in 1918). The two unions amalgamated in 1946 to form the backbone of COHSE. It seems that Nightingale's training methods penetrated the asylums earlier than the poor law institutions.[24] But a large proportion of asylum nurses were men, employed largely for their ability to contain patients physically (in the absence of psychotropic drugs). They were not included in those exclusively feminine Nightingale-style nursing structures that were established, the characteristic pattern being a division both of patients and of nurses into two 'sides' by sex. In view of the expectation attached to men, that they should support their families, it is not surprising to find that they placed more importance than women nurses on pay. Their promotion prospects were relatively poor too. Such were the circumstances that propelled more asylum nurses towards unions in which they joined with other employees, generally of similar or lower status. Unionism was also a more persistent feature among them than among poor law/municipal hospital nurses. Few of the preponderantly female labour force took a sustained interest in power, pay or conditions. Further, the stigmatised asylums, and above all the males who worked there, were as isolated from the bulk of nurses as they could be. However strong the tradition of unionism they built, its influence outside was likely to be negligible. By contrast, poor law nurses were sufficiently exposed to the outward flow of training and example from the larger voluntary hospitals to ally with their non-union tradition. When included, with the National Health Act, in a form of nursing organisation similar to that of the former voluntary hospitals, they tended to follow the lead of the Rcn.

Alongside the industrial unions, 'conglomerate' unions made some inroads among nurses in the 1930s. NALGO was the most successful of these. Interestingly enough, it was not affiliated to the TUC and was viewed as a 'respectable' (predominantly clerical) organisation. As a further indication of the climate within which NALGO members were recruited, we may note that, according to Abel-Smith, most members joined where the matron gave a lead by joining first. It achieved a membership of some 5,000 to 10,000 on paper, though that seems to have been unstable.[25]

Evidently, just as there is division in allegiance between the Rcn and trade unions today, so there was in the 1930s; furthermore, at both times, those nurses who joined were spread among several unions. There is nothing to suggest that membership in the 1930s approached the

current levels; this calls for further examination, centred on the
changing conditions of the struggle.

The Changing Conditions of the Struggle in the 1930s

Nursing is not merely a technical organisation of care for patients,
dictated by the state of the arts; it involves relations of production in
Marx's sense, in which certain interests, in particular medicine and the
state, control others, including nursing. To understand nurses' own
attempts to protect and control their occupation, we must understand
the major changes in these relations of production.

An essential feature of the Nightingale reform was that it created a
unified nursing structure dedicated to 'cleansing' patients and their
environment, both physically and morally. While medicine sought to
'cure', nursing emphasised hygiene and sanitation, and discipline on the
ward. But the subsequent proliferation and expansion of hospitals
favoured the institutionalisation of medicine's curative model.[26] This
led to substantial changes in the content of nursing work and nurses'
relations with other health workers. It has to be borne in mind that
both the nursing structure and the curative model took root most
successfully in the voluntary hospitals. There doctors were able to
attempt cures and could relegate the incurables to public institutions —
the poor law hospitals and asylums. These public institutions were
filled with chronic cases and were relatively impervious both to the
curative model and to Nightingale's reform.

The Nightingale nursing structure was built on social forms that in
the last analysis were in contradiction to those that lay behind the
development of the curative model. It reproduced in the relation
between doctors and nurses the role division between husband and
wife, father and mother, in the bourgeois family. Just as the home
was the province of women, so the hospital ward was the province of
'nurse–housekeepers'. The curative model, however, borrowed not
from gender relations in the wider society but from the organisation of
the factory. Not only did it imply the technical processing of patients'
bodies; it also entailed specialisation among doctors and the
establishment of a division of labour among other health workers,
co-ordinated by the 'doctor–chief-engineer'. In the Nightingale
pattern, nurses formed a relatively autonomous corps with the function
of 'woman' to the doctor's 'man'. Logically, the ascendancy of the
curative model must lead to the breakdown of this corps and the
attachment of individual nurses to medical teams as technical
assistants. The inter-war period in nursing is perhaps fundamentally the

working out in struggle of the contradiction between the nursing structure and the curative model.

Medical specialisation brought in its train the proliferation of ancillary skills: the pharmacist, the X-ray technician and so on. Medicine subordinated these skills.[27] Nurses, who were already working under medical direction, became another ancillary skill or rather a group of skills: they were divided between theatre, general medical, casualty and the rest. Further, as medical mastery of technique grew, so several methods, hitherto considered exclusively medical, were handed down to nurses and other ancillary skills as 'routine'. On receiving these (blood pressures, drips and so on), trained nurses in turn handed down what had hitherto been considered exclusively nursing tasks to lesser-trained or even untrained ward personnel.[28] The most striking instance is the gradual handing down of what Nightingale considered to be the distinctive task of nursing — ward hygiene — until it became a routine practised by 'domestic staff'.

As the technical subordination of nursing developed, so the nursing structure pioneered by the reformers in the larger voluntary hospitals was eroded from within. It was not that the individual nurse was becoming more subordinate, and certainly not that she was losing social status in the eyes of the public. But the structure of domination was changing. In the 'old' pattern, a nurse acted on the orders of the ward sister or matron, even if to service the orders of a doctor: she remained part of a corps in her daily interaction with medicine. In the 'emergent' pattern, she was a technical assistant in one of several rather different teams each commanded by medicine, usually by a single consultant. Further, should a problem on the ward require the services of ancillary professions, the patient was taken from the command of the ward sister, who in the old pattern controlled and co-ordinated all access to the patient (with the partial exception of that of consultants). This incipient erosion of the inner discipline of the nursing corps helps explain the tenacity with which matrons and national leaders in the 1930s defended the matron's control of training, hours of work and even leisure of nurses, and protected from change as best they could a content of training (linked to low pay) which made becoming a nurse an ordeal, a novitiate in humility and rectitude.

As was noted earlier, nursing leadership was pushed at the close of the 1930s to accept the principles of a second portal of entry and to supplant the concept of a unified and homogeneous corps of nurses with the concept of a grade system. First, the growing army of lesser-trained or untrained people doing nursing could be annexed to the corps, as nurses of a lower grade, thus circumventing unionism and evading the threat of dilution of labour. In the event, this second portal of entry (for assistant nurses) proved to be of little significance, though it opened the way for the SEN status. Secondly, however, fully trained nurses could work closely with the doctor as technical assistants (or in his absence perform 'technical' tasks, hitherto medicine's province), while other nursing work, especially 'basic' work, could be handed down to inferior grades acting under the supervision of the trained. Thus the trained nurse could embrace her emergent standing in the technical division of labour and still control basic nursing, even if she did not perform it. This even made possible the retention of the system of training which forced learners to do much of the basic (even the domestic) work of the ward.

As we shall see in the next section, the 'grade system' was to prove an unstable solution to the erosion from within of the internal control of nursing. It could not, of course, prevent the proliferation of medical specialisms and the professional and technical services ancillary to medicine. Not only did the task of co-ordinating all the treatments of her patients slip from the ward sister, but her superiors found that the problem of co-ordinating nurses in many different work-settings called for 'management' skills (i.e. bureaucratic programming). Thus the local leadership in nursing found its base of authority shift from seniority to technical competence or managerial office. Furthermore, at first the lower-grade entrants, and then even students, proved to have experience or commitments outside nursing. The second-level training, like the post of nursing auxiliary, attracted more married women, more people with previous employment, and more who wished to work part-time. Thus the grade system drew within the nursing corps people less susceptible to its disciplines, who had not endured its novitiate. As for the students, the expansion of opportunities for (almost always more lucrative and less arduous) employment for girls was drawing recruitment to low levels even in the late 1930s. When the hospital ceased to be the household of the matron and her corps of nurses, it became more like any other place of employment.

Outside the cure-oriented specialisms that grew up chiefly in the larger voluntary hospitals prior to nationalisation, the pattern of nursing was different at the outset and was not transformed in the same fashion. In Nightingale's time poor law nursing was a species of domestic labour that was carried out by the more able-bodied female paupers on fellow inmates, under the supervision of the lay super-intendent of the workhouse or infirmary.[29] As, under pressure from a few reformers and local medical officers, sickness and the sin of pauperism were slowly disentangled,[30] so began (rather sporadic) experiments with the introduction usually of a single trained nurse, who was to discipline and train other employees or even paupers. Work in these institutions was not attractive to either doctors or nurses with training (and breeding). They were encumbered with the chronic sick and aged, and employment there was confined to local doctors who would accept the small salary and local women who would nurse without training. This situation changed slowly and, when the poor law institutions were taken over by local authorities in the 1930s, they remained less well staffed than voluntary hospitals.[31] Except in the few cases where the reformers made inroads, poor law nurses worked under the supervision at first of the lay superintendent, and then of the medical superintendent of the institution. But the absence of a nursing structure should not blind one to the probability that, individually and as an informal body, nurses in constant attendance on the infirm exercised considerable 'front-line' power, independent of doctors and administrators. Parallel conditions prevailed in the psychiatric sector; though from time to time medicine intervened here, expected cures, containment of patients consistently played a more important part than in any other sector of health care, and in this respect the independent role of the nurse was crucial. These were the distinctive conditions that supported the strength of unionism in the public sector during the 1930s.

The Recent Development of Managerialism in Health Care and its Effect on Nursing

In recent years a new element has entered the context within which nurses' occupational struggles are conducted. The nationalisation of health care in 1948 had a restricted effect on the organisation of hospitals, especially of those that were formerly voluntary. However, from the late 1930s, management structures (and techniques) were introduced to rationalise the distribution and utilisation of resources. The series of changes, which includes the Salmon reform of nursing and the 1974 reorganisation of the NHS as a whole, can only be understood in terms of the logic of state intervention within a class society the dynamic of which is the accumulation of capital.[32]

Parts of industry and commerce — some 'individual capitals' — were to become closely dependent on the growth of high-technology medicine. The profits of drug companies and manufacturers of medical equipment and supplies (such as gases) clearly stood to gain.[33]

However, for capital in general, especially in conditions of recession and/or inflation, a high level of spending on health care may be a liability (regardless of whether it is 'public'). This is because during a recession, or rather on impending recovery from recession, liquidity is at a premium, and the diversion of funds into spheres in which the gain to surplus value is not immediate impedes the economy. Alternatively, in periods of inflation, production as labour intensive as is health care cannot readily be cheapened, and so gets relatively expensive by comparison with more capital-intensive production.[34] Control of health care by the state has the advantage from the standpoint of capital in general that legitimate power can be used to ration supply, whatever the demand, by appealing to 'national interest'. Given the seemingly inexhaustible demand for medical care, it is unlikely that market forces could make these adjustments, certainly in the short term. Hence the paradox that, while the state intervened in health care to support and expand existing provision, it has found itself from time to time seeking to economise or even cut these services.

Since the setting up of the NHS, the state's intervention as 'economiser' has passed from an earlier phase of accountancy control to the present phase of managerialism. As soon as it became apparent (in the 1950s) that the NHS was not going to work itself out of business, but that the demand for care, especially for hospital cures, seemed to expand with supply, the accountant came into his own. Controls were attempted on the amounts spent in different sectors. But the decisive steps from the viewpoint of nursing were taken in the 1960s. Instead of merely holding tight the purse strings, the state sought to evolve new structures of management and work organisation that could achieve economies in the use of resources. The model for these was big business management. Large-scale, geographically far-flung business corporations depended on controlling not only what money was spent, but also how it was spent, in the interests of achieving 'economies of scale' through standardisation and exploiting the best opportunities for profit. The new managerialism of the NHS was developed to minimise costs rather than to make profits, but many of the principles were the same as those used in business. It was argued, for example, that economies could be effected by standardising the purchase of supplies, by centralising services (such as laundry) for several units near to each other, by changing the way work was organised and adopting incentive schemes. Finding economies and implementing them depended upon drawing together at the top the various threads of decision making and committing middle and lower management to following well-defined procedures — so, at least, it was believed.[35]

Part of the introduction of this 'corporate' managerialism was the implementation of the recommendations of the Salmon Report.[36] The implications of this report seemed confusing at the time to nursing. In common with proposals for corporate management in local government and, indeed, in industry, this advertised simultaneously the advantages of centralisation and of devolution. Furthermore, it appeared to open to nursing an extended career hierarchy, and to promise an equal role with medicine and administration in the planning of the hospital. Because technical specialisation within nursing, and the second line of defence (the grade system) adopted by leadership in response to the threat of loss of internal control, had already stratified nursing, the upper strata were readily seduced by the promises. In the event, the Salmon changes, and the wider developments in management that accompanied them, divided nursing between those committed to management and those involved in clinical nursing. Middle managers discovered that their discretion was circumscribed by their heads of department; and heads of department that there always seemed some yet higher authority to whom they were accountable. It is in this context that we have to understand the attitudes of nurses at Westmid towards 'management'. We can characterise it, in a phrase, as the erosion of the grade system by managerialism.

In spite of the differences we have observed in the organisation of work in the 'acute' and geriatric and psychiatric sectors, managerialism was introduced in all sectors. Arguably, it struck at the autonomy of nursing in geriatrics and psychiatry to a degree that medicine had failed to do; further, because of the solidarity their mode of production engendered, nurses here responded to the consciousness of their employment relation, and the conflict of interests with management, by joining the same union as each other, regardless of grade, and building a union culture lacking in the acute hospitals. For example, if we look outside the type of psychiatric unit represented at Westmid to the mental hospitals, it is evident that the late 1960s and the 1970s were marked by two changes. First, a good many hospitals were the subject of high-level inquiries, usually into treatment of patients by nurses.[37] This struck at the relative immunity of staff in these institutions and was the prelude to a period of equivocal state policy towards psychiatric hospitals, in which it was said at one and the same time that mental illness should have higher priority and that more treatment should be provided outside institutions, especially 'in the community'. Little, however, seemed to happen except a steady diminution of the resources available to the hospitals.[38] Secondly, the Salmon proposals were implemented here as elsewhere. The large number of male nurses here, as Carpenter[39] has suggested, have benefited by finding in the new managerial posts opportunities for promotion often blocked in the older arrangement of the two 'sides'. However, these same people and their female counterparts also often took up posts outside their original place of work: the reform of management opened top posts to outsiders. Again, this had the effect of breaching the closure of the institutions and presumably of undermining the informal order that would have grown up as people promoted from within paid their debts to those who had helped them and whom they had left behind. Thus, in mental hospitals, as in the acute sector, the managerial demiurge of recent years has shaken established relations at work and sown the seeds of a rift between rank-and-file nurses and management.

Conclusion: Unionism and the Change in the Mode of Production of Nursing Care

In this chapter we have sought a synoptic view of those changes which brought about the present pattern of struggle by nursing as an occupation. The scope of the inquiry has been dictated by our attempt to adhere to the method of historical materialism, and, within this framework, we have also pointed to the need to conduct studies of the present and of the past in a reciprocal relation to each other. The analysis of the survey of nurses in Westmid AHA guided us to certain lines of inquiry about the past; while, at the same time as this historical analysis has proceeded, it has become clear that the survey findings take their specific significance from changes that have happened over a long period of time, and could scarcely have been observed by a field-worker.

The completeness of membership of organisations that we observed at Westmid, and which seems typical of the country as a whole, probably dates from the dispute of 1974; the degree to which unionism has made inroads among trained nurses is also recent, and even now it is likely that nurses in the teaching hospitals turn to the Rcn rather than trade unions. However, the scatter of membership among professional association and trade unions, and among various unions, has parallels in the 1930s.

We have argued that the scatter of membership in the 1930s was

rooted in contradictions in the market for nursing labour. There was a
rift between the larger voluntary hospitals, employing the greater part
of trained nurses, and the (growing) municipal hospitals and county
mental hospitals, where the untrained were preponderant. When
'nursing leadership', with its base in the larger voluntary hospitals,
conceded to the authorities the principle of a second portal of entry, it
laid the foundations of the 'grade system', which offered the possibility
of control by trained nurses over others involved in nursing.

Nevertheless, the 'leadership' had to struggle against external
intrusions on its control of the market and even of education, by
medicine, the state and the hospitals themselves; it was in a position of
weakness in relation to each, and frequently forced into alliances with
one or another to combat the rest. This, among other things, helps
explain the adamant way in which matrons and the Rcn defended the
old pattern of the 'nursing structure', headed by the matron. Internal
control had to be preserved. The 'grade system' was a second line of
defence.

For its part, unionism was restricted by its very strength among the
excluded, especially among the male nurses of the mental hospitals. To
the preponderant women of the municipal hospitals, and even women
nurses in the mental hospitals, the nursing of the larger voluntary
hospitals was a reference group. Once offered inclusion, especially by
nationalisation, they accepted the leadership of the Rcn.

The significance of this earlier history for the current situation is
twofold. First, it is evident that the rifts and contradictions of the
present have not only parallels but certain continuities with the past.
Thus there remain divisions in memberships between upper-grade and
lower-grade nurses and between those in the 'acute' (medical/surgical)
sector, as represented here by the Westmid Infirmary and in the 1930s
by the larger voluntary hospitals, and those in the psychiatric and
'chronic' sectors, here the city hospital and earlier the municipal
hospitals and county mental hospitals. Secondly, just as the spurt of
unionism in the 1930s reflected the inability of the 'nursing structure'
to control nursing as a whole and was eclipsed by the advent of a new
system of internal control — the 'grade system' — so, we would argue,
the new unionism reflects the collapse of the 'grade system' and the
failure of nursing to evolve (at least as yet) a new structure of internal
control appropriate to the emergent conditions.

To this point our historical analysis has been all but confined to the
'politics' of nursing in the inter-war period and up to the National
Health Act. In this, except for some quite marked differences of

interpretation (particularly in the use of the notion of 'contradiction' and of conceptual frameworks for analysing unionism and professionalism), it resembles Abel-Smith's deservedly acknowledged work and indeed hangs heavily upon it. We clearly part company with him when we insist that the occupational strategies of nursing must be understood ultimately in terms of changes in the 'mode of production of nursing care'.

This is the shift of focus most distinctive of historical materialism. But this mode of production must not be understood as if merely a piece of 'technology' — a woman—organisation—machine/tool combination. It is built from the social forms available in its epoch, whether these be class and gender relations, forms of work organisation in industry or the pattern of 'corporate management'. In this way 'social history' becomes of direct and pressing relevance to the history of nursing, not as a backcloth to events on stage, but as the constitutive rules of the script itself.

We have tentatively broken down the major epochs in the mode of production of nursing care into three phases. In the first, lady nurses acted as hospital housekeepers, but as members of a disciplined corps rather than individual professionals, alongside doctors, who were emerging as individual professionals. Nightingale founded this mode, and it lived on into the inter-war period, being superseded only in the second war and its aftermath. It was rooted in the class and gender relations of late Victorian England.

The second phase began in the period between the wars, was marked by the contradiction between the respective social forms on which the nursing structure and the curative model were built, and was what lay behind the crisis of internal control that characterised the behaviour of nursing leadership and came to a head in the late 1930s. It was marked by the subordination of nursing to medicine within a technical division of labour, in which several other occupations were joined. This change depended on the second industrial revolution — in particular, the example of engineering, both in mechanics and in chemicals, and the extension of 'engineering' principles to management of people — and also upon the confidence now reposed by the bourgeoisie in 'hospital cures'. It was an uneven change, that is still in motion (though now, at the 'hot' end, increasingly dependent on the third industrial revolution, in electronics). Only recently has the intervention of medicine in psychiatry and geriatrics become at all marked, and differences in the current pattern of membership of organisations by nurses may well reflect the relative autonomy of nursing as a body in these specialisms.

The third phase was marked by state intervention. State mediation, even in the relation between doctor and patient, reached back to the inter-war period, but began to climb to its current peak in the late 1960s. In this context, it was dictated by the drive to economise in public spending. The model of 'corporate management' that was currently available from the dominant sphere of corporate monopoly capitalism was adopted in the hospitals as in many other public institutions. The effect was to split management from workers, even in nursing, as was dramatically evident at Westmid from the alignment of management with the Rcn and clinical nurses with unions, and from the tendency of clinical nurses to look to their local union officers for mediation in matters of discipline with a management perceived now as 'remote'. The second phase prepared much of the ground for the split between grades in nursing, and its uneven development explained the eventual scatter of membership among various organisations. But the managerialism of the third phase laid the foundations for the unprecedented rise in numbers joining unions, especially among trained nurses at clinical level. Clinical nurses now focused their attention on the employment relation — on factors such as pay, power and working conditions. Inflation, the successful unionism of ancillary workers and the new militancy of junior doctors in the mid-1970s were only the catalysts of a reaction formed from ingredients already provided.

Notes

1. M. Foucault, *Discipline and Punish* (Allen Lane, Harmondsworth, 1977), p. 31.

2. J. Goody and I. Watt, 'The Consequences of Literacy', in P. Giglioli (ed.), *Language and Social Context* (Penguin, Harmondsworth, 1972), pp. 316–18.

3. E.g. E. R. Bendall and E. Raybould, *A History of the General Nursing Council for England and Wales: 1919–1969* (H. K. Lewis, London, 1970).

4. R. White, *Social Change and the Development of the Nursing Profession* (Henry Kimpton, London, 1978).

5. F. R. Adam, 'From Association to Union: professional organisation of Asylum Attendants, 1869–1919', *British Journal of Sociology*, vol. 20 (1969), pp. 11–26.

6. P. Bellaby and P. Oribabor, 'The growth of trade union consciousness among general hospital nurses', *Sociological Review*, vol. 25, new series (1977), pp. 801–22.

7. See, especially, K. Marx and F. Engels, *The German Ideology*, Part 1 (Lawrence and Wishart, London, 1968); and K. Marx, 'Preface, Contribution to a Critique of Political Economy', in Marx and Engels, *Selected Works* (Lawrence and Wishart, London, 1968), pp. 181–5.

8. For a general discussion along these lines, see L. Colletti, *Marx and Hegel* (New Left Books, London, 1973).

9. Such as V. I. Lenin, *The Development of Capitalism in Russia* (Progress Publishers, Moscow, 1956); K. Marx, 'On primitive accumulation', in *Capital*, vol. 1, Part 8 (Penguin, Harmondsworth, 1976).

10. For further analysis see P. Oribabor, 'The Organisation of Work and the Occupational Strategy of Hospital Nurses', unpublished PhD thesis, University of Keele, 1979. We should like to express our gratitude to all those who collaborated in the study. The analysis was done with the aid of the SPSS system and we are particularly grateful to Paul Collis of the Computer Centre, Keele, for his advice. The project was funded by a studentship from the SSRC.

11. 'Completeness' and 'character' are the concepts of R. A. Blackburn, *Union Character and Social Class: a study of White Collar Unionism* (Batsford, London, 1967), see Introductory Chapter.

12. Also of a dispute among organisations representing nurses. COHSE mounted several one-day stoppages, which both NUPE and the Rcn regretted. However, the Rcn threatened mass resignation from the NHS. The dispute was resolved by the Halsbury Report.

13. R. Hyman and I. Brough, *Social Values and Industrial Relations* (Blackwell, Oxford, 1975).

14. Oribabor, 'Hospital Nurses'.

15. The proportions of the Westmid sample (including nursing officers) who were Rcn and NUPE members respectively are similar to those claimed nationally by the organisations at about that time (in June 1977 the Rcn had 90,000 members; and, according to S. S. Lewis, 'Nurses and Trade Unions in Britain', *International Journal of Health Services*, vol. 6, 4 (1976), pp. 641–9, NUPE had 80,000 nurse members in 1976). However, NALGO was almost certainly more successful at Westmid than nationally, and COHSE less so. Neither NALGO nor COHSE requires its branches to break down membership by category of staff. In correspondence, Mick Carpenter has suggested that NALGO may have only 10,000 nurse members across the country, while COHSE may have almost as many as other organisations put together (170,000 – though this figure seems to us doubtful, because COHSE's total membership is only 250,000). More reliable figures may be produced from analysis of subscriptions deducted from salary, which, we gather, Roger Dyson is shortly to undertake for one region. Since the winter of 1977/78, when the Westmid survey was conducted, there has been some shift of membership in the Rcn's favour, especially following NUPE's strike action in the winter of 1978/79. The Rcn currently (June 1979) claims 150,000 members.

16. B. Abel-Smith, *A History of the Nursing Profession* (Heinemann, London, 1960), pp. 143–4.

17. Abel-Smith, *Nursing Profession*, Ch. XI.

18. T. Johnson, *Professions and Power* (Macmillan, London, 1972).

19. D. Klegon, 'The sociology of professions: an emerging perspective', *Sociology of Work and Occupations*, vol. 5, 3 (August 1978).

20. W. Hector, *Mrs. Bedford Fenwick* (Rcn, London, 1973).

21. Abel-Smith, *Nursing Profession*, pp. 181–90.

22. To add substance to this point, we may note that, though the initial reaction of nursing leadership to the Wood Committee was hostile, by the 1950s it had adopted aspects of the Wood proposals as its own. There are several instances of a similar kind in nursing history. See C. Davies, 'Four Events in Nursing History: A New Look', *Nursing Times Occasional Papers*, vol. 74 (1978).

23. R. Hyman, *Industrial Relations: A Marxist Introduction* (Macmillan, London, 1975).

24. M. Carpenter, 'The New Managerialism and Professionalism in Nursing', in

M. Stacey *et al.* (eds), *Health and The Division of Labour* (Croom Helm, London, 1977). See also Carpenter in this volume.

25. Abel-Smith, *Nursing Profession*, pp. 142–3.

26. T. McKeown, *Medicine in Modern Society* (Allen and Unwin, London, 1965).

27. C. A. Brown, 'The division of labour: allied health professions', *International Journal of Health Services*, vol. 3, 3 (1973).

28. E. A. Krause, *Power and Illness* (Elsevier, New York, 1977), Ch. 1.

29. B. Abel-Smith, *The Hospitals 1800–1948* (Heinemann, London, 1964).

30. R. Hodgkinson, *The Origin of the National Health Service: The Medical Services of the Poor Law 1834–1871* (Wellcome Institute of the History of Medicine, London, 1967). See also Dean and Bolton in this volume.

31. J. Willcocks, *The Creation of the National Health Service: A Study of Pressure Group and a Major Social Policy Decision* (Routledge, London, 1967).

32. For a more extended discussion see P. Bellaby and P. Oribabor, 'Determinants of the occupational strategies of British hospital nurses', *International Journal of Health Services*, 10 (1980); and V. Navarro, *Class Struggle, the State and Medicine: A Historical and Contemporary Analysis of the Medical Sector in Great Britain* (Martin Robertson, London, 1978).

33. H. B. Myers, 'The medical-industrial complex', *Fortune*, 81 (January 1970).

34. B. Fine and L. Harris, 'The debate on state expenditure', *New Left Review*, 98 (1976), p. 105; I. Gough, 'State expenditure in advanced capitalism', *New Left Review*, 92 (1975).

35. J. D. Stewart, 'Programme budgetting in British Local Government', *Local Government Finance* (November 1969), pp. 454–66. See also C. Whittington and P. Bellaby, 'The reasons for hierarchy in Social Services Departments', *Sociological Review*, vol. 27, new series (1979), pp. 513–49.

36. Ministry of Health and Scottish Home and Health Department, Report of the Committee on Senior Nursing Staff Structure (Salmon) (HMSO, London, 1966). See also Carpenter, 'New Managerialism', pp. 175–8.

37. For instance: DHSS, Report of the Committee of Inquiry into allegations of ill-treatment of patients and other irregularities at the Ely Hospital, Cardiff (HMSO, 1969); DHSS, Report of the Committee of Inquiry into Whittingham Hospital (HMSO, 1972); South-East Thames Regional Health Authority, Report of the Committee of Inquiry into the care and treatment of patients at St Augustine's Hospital, Chartham, Canterbury (1976).

38. P. Townsend, 'Inequality and the Health Services', *The Lancet* (June 1974), p. 1179.

39. Carpenter, 'New Managerialism', p. 181.

8 OLD WIVES' TALES? WOMEN HEALERS IN ENGLISH HISTORY

Margaret Connor Versluysen

Should we be studying nursing history at all? This is the question, a
fundamental one, raised here by Margaret Connor Versluysen. She sees
existing history as history from a male viewpoint — a viewpoint which
has devalued and trivialised women's work. She shows that there is
alternative material, though it is not often noticed, on women healers,
and argues that this deserves a much more central place in our
attention. The work of two authors, Ehrenreich and English, who have
raised questions in this field, is assessed here. This work is frankly
polemical; it is not a work of detailed historical scholarship. But such
works, Versluysen argues, have a place in rewriting history, in
sketching out a more adequate theoretical position from which we can
begin.

What kind of work should we be doing, if we take this analysis
seriously? Certainly, for some, it means starting further back than the
nineteenth century and asking about, not taking for granted, the sexual
divisions which became established then. Others need to build into their
work an analysis of the differential treatment of men and women.
Carpenter in this volume has begun to do just this for asylum nurses.
Undeniably, a major problem now and in the past is that so many
nurses are women, that we have not got comparative cases and that we
fail to see and appreciate the difference this makes. Critiques such as
this can help keep us alert.

—————Ed.

In a statistical sense women have always been the main healers in
English society. They have delivered babies, rendered first aid,
prescribed and dispensed remedies and cared for the sick, infirm and
dying, both as a neighbourly service and as paid work. Yet, aside from
histories of nursing, the vast range of women's past healing work is
virtually absent from the annals of written history.

This chapter will claim that this is due to biases about women which
are embedded in the basic frame of reference of history. Our task here
will be to make explicit some of the implicit sexual biases in the
historical literature. This will show how uncritical value judgements
about the sexes have induced historians to ignore a great deal of
potential data about women's role in the social management of health
and illness. Secondly, little-known work of feminist scholars will be
cited, providing evidence of extensive female healing roles in the past
very different from those we know today. This evidence suggests that

175

conventional distinctions between doctoring and nursing, amateur and professional medicine, orthodox and unorthodox healers may be less relevant for an analysis of the past than distinctions between men and women. This critique should inform our evaluation of existent histories and will raise an agenda of potential research problems for the future. To develop this critique we must begin with some definition of history as an intellectual enterprise, in order to see how and why the methods of historical research have predisposed the discipline to ignore or devalue the predecessors of today's nurses, midwives and female health workers.

What is History?

History is not the past *per se*, but is primarily an intellectual operation which reconstructs the past through the interpretation of fragmentary written residues. Historical study is intrinsically selective in several senses. First, the historian can only draw upon available sources. These are usually what long-dead men and women have themselves seen as worthy of written record. Secondly, the historian selects that which seems relevant from a sampling of the sources and interprets the findings in accordance with her/his own social values and intellectual schema. Since historical data can only be gathered and sifted on the basis of some prior intellectual assumptions and categories held by the historian, it follows that an historian necessarily holds some implicit values and theories about the data, however ill defined or unformulated they may be. Hence history is always both selective and value laden and can never be an atheoretical, neutral collection of 'facts', since 'facts' only become history via the intervention of individual historians. Thus history is 'objective' only in the sense that the historian dispassionately presents the analysis and findings in such a way that they are amenable to critical scrutiny by other scholars.

Despite the scholarly detachment most historians have brought to their work, there is a third very significant sense in which history has been highly selective, indeed one-dimensional. To date, most history has addressed the past solely from the point of view of men, male interests, values and concerns. Our legacy is a literature in which vast tracts of the past seem to have been populated (quite remarkably) exclusively by men! Sometimes we catch sight of female shadows in the distance, but the devaluation and trivialisation of women's lives and concerns have usually meant that sustained systematic study of women's past has been ruled out of the historical court. Recent growth of interest in the history of childhood, the family and related topics is beginning to provide some fragmentary information about women. Feminist scholarship is slowly pinpointing women's interests on the map of history.[1] But this is a tiny drop in a vast ocean of disinterest and apathy. Moreover, the consistency and thoroughness with which history has either ignored or devalued the study of women are not purely accidental.

History, like the other academic professions, is male dominated and its value system is overwhelmingly male. Historians, like other social groups, derive many of their values and beliefs from those which are dominant in the society in which they live and work. Beliefs and ideas produced in the environing society are incorporated into historical orthodoxies, where they provide agreed-upon criteria which infuse the scholarly community's approach to its own work. If history has failed to study women as it has studied men, and has treated the sexes unequally, it has simply reflected the principal values and social arrangements of a sexually unequal society. Our society has evolved an elaborate set of beliefs to justify its consistent ranking and rewarding of male interests and activities more highly than comparable female interests and activities. This belief system has usually informed historical investigation and explanation. If we look into the mirror of history, we find a systematic interpretation of past health care practice in a way which assigns positive value and superior status to male healing work, and little or no value and subordinate or marginal status to female activity.[2] But, as we shall see, this is only one interpretation of the past, and not a representation of any absolute historical truth.

Great Men and Invisible Women: Myths and Stereotypes

To date, the history of health care has been fairly narrowly conceived as the history of organised medicine. Organised medicine, especially its most prestigious branches, has formally barred women from its ranks for most of its known past. History has reflected this sexual exclusivity and has been primarily the story of a socially privileged group of male healers. Moreover, within these limited parameters, there has been an even narrower preoccupation with the role of medical ideas as agents of social progress. This has led to the dominance in history of an heroic 'great men of medicine' theory of medical development and social change. Hence the history of the health field has been seen primarily as that of the ideas and discoveries of 'great men' of medicine carrying the tide of health knowledge to its present state of sophistication and complexity.

This sort of view is intimately bound up with the idea of history as intrinsically progressive, since it assumes that society is constantly evolving to higher and ever more rational forms of organisation. This assumption is only possible because it is premised on a belief that society is egalitarian and that change will include and benefit everyone regardless of class or sex. But whatever real debt we owe to great physicians of the past, these few individuals did not make history alone, nor has the development of our contemporary health care system resulted solely from the supposed triumph of male medical rationality over the supposedly non-rational superstitions of some male quacks and a mass of illiterate 'old wives'. That is, at the very least, a sexually selective and extremely partial view of the past.

Moreover, male medical ideas and values have been the main yardstick against which historians have measured potential topics chosen for investigation and formulated types of questions asked of the historical data and the categories used to evaluate raw materials from the past. Traditionally, the medical men have dismissed any personnel or ideas falling outside their own domain of control as of little significance or consequence. Historians have generally accepted this dismissal with great alacrity and little criticism. Until well into the nineteenth century, other healers frequently competed with medical men for custom. An essential part of the medical armoury against this competition was a self-aggrandising rhetoric which depicted all other healers as irregular, unorthodox, amateurs or quacks. This usually went hand in hand with the medical groups' claims to unique jurisdiction over, or special expertise in, certain therapies and techniques,[3] however ill founded those claims may have been. Historians have generally accepted this medical view, and readily dismissed non-medical personnel as mere amateurs who were quite marginal to the maintenance of the physical health and well-being of society. This is an extremely limited value judgement, since before the eighteenth century there were very few doctors except in a handful of urban centres. Hence the management of birth, child-rearing, illness, infirmity and death was, for the majority of the population, in the hands of 'amateurs'. The majority of these unspecified 'amateurs' were women, whom the medical profession and historical convention have suggested were simply a mass of illiterate old wives who caused more illness than they ever prevented or cured.

We will contest this old wife mythology later. In the meantime it is
enough to note that what most historians have ignored, or dismissed as
amateur domestic medicine, was an extensive system of home-based
health care. In this country almost all medieval hospitals were destroyed
by the Reformation and, before the growth of voluntary hospitals and
dispensaries from the eighteenth century and poor law infirmaries from
the nineteenth century, healing took place primarily in the healer's or
patient's own home, and is therefore not easily observable. But a wide
range of sources exists as a testament to women's past healing practice
– diaries, memoirs, letters, housewifery manuals, herbal compendia,
popular health manuals, and local records and archives, to name but a
few. Many of these mention female healing work, whilst popular works
on health and illness were frequently addressed to women or, as in the
case of midwifery texts, were often written by women. Yet this
potential evidence has hardly been tapped, since historians have
assumed, quite incorrectly, that women's healing work constitutes the
mere trivia of history. Historians' reverence for the male medical view
has induced them to prefer source material from a medical pen. Many
past medical writers had some vested interest in the derogation of
women's healing skills, especially in periods when doctors and women
competed for clientele.[4] This suggests a very simple hypothesis – i.e.
that there may be some causal connection between medical misogyny
and the closure of medical occupations to women. A recent
feminist study of seventeenth-century medicine advances arguments
which could lend weight to this hypothesis.[5] More seriously, however,
historians have often accepted pejorative value judgements about
women healers' work, as if these were statements of proven historical
fact. Usually they were not. Furthermore, in relying primarily on
medical writings and records, historians have ignored other sources
which put a positive rather than a negative value on women's healing
work. Hence, we can take history to task for its highly selective
sampling of available material and biased reading of data.

Not that history has ignored women's existence completely; often it
has employed a far more subtle, if powerful, convention, which we are
familiar with from everyday life, namely the stereotyping of all women
by exaggerating certain individual characteristics which are believed to
be especially 'feminine'. In health care history women have appeared
mainly in a triptych of stereotypes as illiterate old wives, exceptional
wives, exceptional heroines or saintly ministering angels whose mystical
aura contrasts starkly with the apparent rationality of male medicine.
These images are by definition one-sided exaggerations which tell us

about social attitudes to women rather than contribute any valid systematic historical knowledge about women healers as a social collectivity. Whether these images are romantically flattering or negatively misogynist, this stereotyped individualisation of female healing virtually denies the evidence of a wide-spread healing role for the female sex. Even the relatively heroic, romantic accounts of nursing saints, nineteenth-century reformers and pioneer female physicians hardly redress the balance. By definition, the study of a few exceptional women is a study of the unrepresentative and atypical, and simply lends weight to the mistaken belief that, aside from these few notable individuals, the female sex as a whole was marginal rather than integral to rational care of the sick. Even in nursing history, the prototypical female healing occupation, we find that a few heroic women have been singled out, whilst the bulk of the past nursing labour force has been condemned to obscurity as effectively as if, like the fictitious 'Sarah Gamp', it had never existed at all. If rank-and-file nurses have elicited little interest, what of nursing heroines? Even these, it seems, have generally been fitted into some pre-given mould which accords with biases about expected female behaviour. Florence Nightingale, the nursing heroine *par excellence*, is a salient example. The Nightingale literature has too often presented this remarkable woman as a stereotype within a stereotype.[6]

After the Crimea, Nightingale became an immediate myth amongst her contemporaries, attracting more than fifty biographers, many of them in her own lifetime. Predictably, the majority of these preferred to concentrate on her relatively brief time in the Crimea as the 'Lady with the Lamp' or on her work as the 'Founder of Modern Nursing'. But these were minor facets of a remarkable life. Nightingale's more significant historical achievements as pioneer medical statistician, radical reformer of the British Army Medical Corps, political expert on Imperial India and architect of the massive Indian Sanitary Commission have elicited much less attention and interest, presumably because these roles do not fit conveniently into the legend of ministering angel and drawing-room reformer, the expected stereotypes of a Victorian lady; i.e. Nightingale's real intellectual achievements conflict with myths about femininity. For a myth is not built on untruth, but rather on a highly selective interpretation of facts, and the Nightingale literature 'presents a classic case study of the transmission of an historical myth'.[7]

The history of the nursing occupation as a whole has not attracted more than a handful of serious scholars.[8] Historians' focus on exceptional women accounts for remarkable gaps in our knowledge about the nursing past, even in the relatively well-mined nineteenth century. The largest single group of nurses in regular public employment in this period – in the poor law service – have only just been rescued from the workhouse. In a recent book, White does much to rehabilitate the image of the poor law nursing service by showing that its members were not necessarily drunken incompetents nor passive uncaring ciphers, but often achieved relatively high standards of nursing care, and sometimes championed the cause of their chronically sick patients in the face of a less than sympathetic officialdom.[9]

Although the survival of the species depends upon the successful management of childbirth, historical interest in midwifery and birth customs has been almost non-existent. Perhaps this is because birth has always been regarded as 'women's business', and was not formally included in organised medicine until the end of the nineteenth century.[10] But female midwifery had a long genealogy and was one of the few female occupations which had formal recognised public status in the pre-medical era. We can trace records of royal midwives back to the fifteenth century, whilst ecclesiastical licensing of 'professed' midwives began in the sixteenth century. Despite considerable source material, the first comprehensive social history of English midwives was not published until 1977.[11] Prior to this, although one does encounter favourable references to continental midwifery schools, one must generally search through medical histories of past childbirth practices for dismissive or pejorative allusions to English midwives. The only other work which approaches the scale and depth of the 1977 study was published by an obstetrician, J. H. Aveling, in 1872.[12] This conveys the impression that rationally managed childbirth was the sole invention of the medical profession. It is possible to interpret the historical data very differently, but this has rarely been done.[13] Why? Primarily because myths about superior male rationality and expertise over female ignorance and incompetence are so deeply entrenched that they are rarely questioned or criticised. Hence, the myths live on in history and in the society that sustains its work.

Nursing History and 'Petticoat Physic'

In 1881 no less an authority than Nightingale herself insisted that 'To be a good nurse one must be a good woman', which for nurses meant '*attendants* on the Wants of the Sick – *helpers* in carrying out Doctors' orders'.[14] Ever since, the equation woman = nurse = attendant = medical helpmate has dominated society's view of the position and roles of women in the healing process. This service role is usually believed to coincide with women's 'natural' biological functions, since supposedly women intrinsically possess expressive, maternal, caring qualities especially appropriate to the care of the sick. By contrast, the male medical profession is seen as the scientific head of patient care; nurses and other women engaged in the womanly business of caring are merely its maternal heart. As a 1905 edition of *Hospital* expressed it: 'Ability to care for the helpless is women's distinctive nature. Nursing is mothering. Grown up folks when very sick are all babies.'[15] If women have baulked at the limitations of this role, and have wanted to develop diagnostic and other skills conventionally seen as 'masculine', they have been told they were rejecting their very 'feminine' natures. As a feminist scholar has pointed out:

> One thing that emerges from the history of the struggle of women to enter the medical profession, is that male doctors of the period were in general more impressed by dogma (about women) than evidence. If women demonstrated they were intellectually equal to men by walking off with the examination prizes, then the reaction was to take the prizes away from them and continue pretending they were inferior, as the editor of the Lancet assured them was the case: 'Woman as a nurse is the natural help of man as a doctor. Woman as a doctor is a conceit contradictory to nature . . .'[16]

It is now a century since women won the battle to enter medicine, but flimsy biologistic arguments about female nature did not die out with reactionary nineteenth-century physicians. Rather, the argument has been reproduced quite regularly in studies of the nursing role which is still seen as intrinsically feminine.[17] But the very narrowly defined and limited service role of the modern nurse, however technologically sophisticated, contrasts sharply with the variety of healing tasks and functions which women undertook before the nineteenth century. This point was made rather forcibly by Sophia Jex Blake, one of the first women to win the battle for acceptance into the modern British medical profession. Jex Blake and her female colleagues faced virulent opposition to what was then derisorily called 'petticoat physic'.

In 1886, she published a short and illuminating treatise in which she appealed to the past to show that women had practised as doctors since ancient times and had made significant contributions to the

advance of medical understanding. Hence, as Jex Blake told her
opponents, there seemed to be no valid historical or biological reason
why she or any other woman should not do the same, apart from the
irrational sexual prejudice of the male establishment.[18] Jex Blake's
claims about women's past efforts in physic and surgery, although
intended to further the political cause of herself and her beleaguered
colleagues, were certainly grounded in historical fact. Indeed, Jex
Blake's theme and the complex genealogy of 'petticoat physic' were
successively taken up by Alice Clark in 1919 in a pioneering study of
women's work, by the medievalist Eileen Power in 1921, by the
American physician historian Kate Campbell Hurd-Mead in 1938 and
finally, in 1943, by Muriel Joy Hughes who focused on the medieval
period in England.[19] These scholars drew on an array of sources which
showed that women's past medical work had been varied and extensive
in scope and had involved women of all social classes, from the wise
women skilled in the use of herbs and ointments, to the chatelaine in
her castle, and the woman selling her skills as physician and surgeon in
the open market. Indeed, material on women's past medical work is
remarkably extensive and a considerable bibliography on the subject
was recently collated and published.[20] This array of evidence suggests
not only that we can regard much of the old wife mythology with some
scepticism, but also that it is quite false to assume that women are
capable of little else but the simplest nursing.

Hurd-Mead traces women's involvement in medicine and surgery
from the Ancient World, through medieval Europe and England up to
the late eighteenth century; Hughes and Power concentrate on the
medieval period, and Clark on seventeenth-century England. Hughes
draws from both literary and medical sources to examine women's
healing effort from the eleventh to the fifteenth century. She claims
that the main responsibility for the administration of medical aid in
this period fell upon women, who nursed the sick, rendered first aid
and attended to servants and guests at home as well as in secular and
conventual hospitals. Healing duties fell so obviously within the sphere
of women and were naturally so accepted in much contemporary
writing. Although women were excluded from the front ranks of
medicine, Hughes paints a remarkable picture of highly literate
educated ladies and fictional heroines, growing medicinal herbs,
dispensing remedies, healing wounded knights, setting bones and
managing the health needs of their communities. Hughes stresses that,
although her data mainly refer to upper-class ladies, women of the
humbler classes were usually skilled in herbal medicine and had learned

the healing arts as best they could from their mothers and other female kin. Furthermore, female healers seem to have been remarkably successful in the multiplicity of healing functions they performed. Hughes says that, despite the attitudes of professional physicians, women's skill in the relief of suffering was widely recognised and contrasted favourably with that of their male rivals. The ministrations of medieval women to the sick were sufficiently successful to win them gratitude, devotion and respect from their contemporaries; female healers were romanticised and glamorised in medieval literature and were attributed almost magical properties.

Power's concern is rather different. In a brief piece she attempts to trace 'something more closely approaching a professional practice of medicine and surgery by women in the Middle Ages', by which she seems to mean women earning their living as doctors. She cites the 'legend of lady doctors at Salerno . . . which was widespread through Europe in the thirteenth century' and examines a famous trial of a woman doctor in Paris, at which eight witnesses were called by the Paris Medical Faculty, 'who could testify that she had used . . . methods of diagnosis and treatment, that she was considered a wise physician, and that she had successfully cured them'. Ironically, the Medical Faculty's objection seems precisely to have been that, although Felicie Jacoba, the accused, had not been licensed by the Faculty, she used similar medical methods and had achieved a considerable reputation and success as a physician. Power offers little evidence about England, except a plaint for a licence to practise from an English woman doctor, and a subsequent edict of the English Parliament of 1421, which includes the clause that 'no woman use the practice of Fisyk, under the same payne (of long emprisonment)'.[21] This petition, which had been brought to Parliament by the physicians, certainly suggests that a considerable number of women had been practising; if they had not, why should this edict have been issued? Clark's work on the later period suggests that, at least up to the seventeenth century, many women continued the practice of medicine undisturbed, despite some persecution by medical guilds trying to enforce their privileges. Clark says that, though we may find many references to women who practised medicine and surgery as a profession, in the majority of cases their skill was used only for the assistance of their family and neighbours.

Women practised medicine and surgery mainly as domestic arts; indeed they were expected to do so. A housekeeping manual of 1700 stresses that women should 'have a competent knowledge of Physick and Chyrugery that they may be able to help their maimed, sick and indigent Neighbours: for Commonly all good and Charitable Ladies make this a part of their housekeeping business'.[22] But women also performed these tasks as paid work, aside from the ancient craft of midwifery; account books of boroughs and parishes show that the poor received medical treatment from men and women. Independent and financially successful female practitioners of medicine and surgery are cited by Clark, who drew on memoirs, letters and family and local archives for her evidence.

Clark and Power were both preoccupied with the extent to which women were paid or not for their healing services, since payment was seen as indicative of some sort of 'professional' standing in the community. However, this criterion may be less relevant than the sheer extent of women's unpaid healing work in a mainly rural pre-market society where ladies of quality willingly gave their services to kin, dependants and the poor for the greater glory of God, and the female community as a whole seems to have been characterised by a considerable degree of mutual aid and support. In fact, other evidence would suggest that, in England before the seventeenth century, women provided healing services, including much now regarded as 'medical', for the vast majority of the population, if only because the family was the main arena for care and because male healers, even those who regarded themselves as medical practitioners, were very few in number. The university-educated physicians of the Royal College were a tiny elite who deliberately restricted their numbers to only 34 members in 1618, a mere fraction of the numbers of practitioners at large,[23] whilst urban-based groups of organised male 'empirics' — i.e. the apothecaries, druggists and barber surgeons — were very small and did not begin to multiply rapidly until the seventeenth and eighteenth centuries.[24]

Such evidence means it is quite possible to suggest that, before the late seventeenth century, the male impact on the everyday healing experience of most people was minimal, especially if it is considered that midwifery and the care of infants and children were exclusively female preserves. In terms of the autonomy of their practice, evident expertise and sheer numbers, women in the past probably were society's unofficial health care experts. If this is so, which is certainly where the evidence points, then it is clear that there is no real basis for the assumption that medical functions — i.e. diagnosis, prescription of therapy and supervision of the sick — are in any sense intrinsically 'masculine' tasks, although the medical profession has often depicted this work as unsuitable for women.

Conventional medical history would suggest that women were

excluded from organised medicine because of their lack of orthodox knowledge and training as compared to men, and hence their unreliable ideas and dangerous practices. But this is a dubious argument on a number of counts, attempting to rationalise female exclusion from medicine, but by no means explaining it satisfactorily. First, history has often assumed a coherence and homogeneity of the medical group, which certainly did not obtain before the unification of the medical profession in the mid-nineteenth century. Before this, the most striking thing about the medical occupation — i.e. the physicians, barber surgeons and apothecaries — was the sheer diversity of their skills, class and educational backgrounds. Before the 1858 Medical Registration Act few medical men, aside from physicians possessed university degrees; surgeons were regarded as craftsmen and apothecaries are tradesmen. Many of these had served an apprenticeship, but the unqualified were legion. Even at the beginning of the nineteenth century, it was still possible to obtain medical qualifications from no less than 18 different, independent licensing bodies, and to purchase illicit medical degrees from less salubrious sources, or simply to hang out a sign calling oneself a doctor. This situation obtained widely until the standardisation of entry to the medical profession in the Medical Registration Act of 1858.[25] Prior to 1858, the physicians had derided and persecuted other medical men, especially the apothecaries, but it is important to understand that, when the profession formally unified in 1858, most of these male groups were incorporated into it with the physicians, whereas women were not. If sex were not the main criterion of professional membership, it would be necessary to explain why certain categories of relatively uneducated men were included in the profession, whilst more highly educated upper-class women were not. Twenty-one years later the reformed profession ceded to pressure from women who wanted to qualify as doctors.[26]

Secondly, female healers are usually alleged to have gained their knowledge in a very casual haphazard manner. But knowledge of healing, like other domestic skills, was passed down from mother to daughter. It was not uncommon for widows to take over their husbands' barber surgeons' or apothecaries' practices, whilst some professed midwives in London had served a seven-year apprenticeship or had trained in a continental school like the Hôtel Dieu. Further, although women may have lacked formal licences, their common sense and evident experience are often compared by contemporaries to the inexperience of doctors. Although the physicians may have been preoccupied with the status of women's skills, Power, Hughes and Clark suggest that patients usually had considerable confidence in women healers' abilities, even if jealous physicians did not. Clark sums up the situation in this way:

> The general standard of efficiency among men who professed medicine and surgery was very low, the chief work of the country practitioner being the letting of blood, and the wise woman of the village may easily have been his superior in other forms of treatment.[27]

She gives a variety of examples of contemporary patients' views.

Thomas Hobbes, the philosopher, 'preferred an experienced old woman' to 'the most learned and inexperienced physician'. The noted oculist, Dr Turbeville, reported that 'he expected to learn something of these Court doctors, but to his amazement he found them only spies upon his practice . . . ; nay farther, he knew several midwives and old women whose advice he would rather follow than theirs'. Sir Ralph Verney advised his wife to give their sick child 'no phisick but such as midwives and old women with the doctors' approbation do prescribe; for assure yourselfe, they by experience know better than any phisition how to treat such infants'.[28] Further, it should be remembered that, despite a long history of medical discovery, it was not until the end of the nineteenth century that male medicine could claim any rigorously scientific orthodoxy for its therapy; before this, medical decisions were often based on extremely arbitrary and conflicting theories of disease causation. Therefore, it is extremely dubious to impute standardised knowledge and expertise to the medical group and mere superstition and ignorance to female practitioners. Evidently, there were both skilled, experienced doctors and some ignorant old wives, but the point is not to prove one or the other but simply to show the falsity of making unconditional generalised assumptions which oversimplify the merits and skills of either sex.

But what of the imputed eternal unchanging link between female nature and nursing the sick? Is there any historical basis for it? Indeed there is not. Healing roles are not static but change through time and have been typed along sex lines in particular ways in specific historical periods; i.e. the designation of certain skills and therapies as 'nursing' responsibilities, and their concomitant allocation to women, is a relatively recent historical product of social change, as we can show if we begin our inquiry in the late medieval period.

Before the seventeenth century, amongst the then limited range of therapeutic interventions, there was little formal distinction between what were thought of as 'doctoring' and 'nursing' tasks. The main differentiation was between classical academic medicine and the work of those outside its domain, i.e. women, and male healers usually referred to as 'empirics', i.e. the barber surgeons, apothecaries, grocers and druggists. Medieval secular and religious nursing orders were either male or female in composition and, apart from midwifery and wet-nursing, it was not until the seventeenth century that a poorly paid low-status area of employment began to emerge on a wide scale and was progressively allocated to women. We can only guess at the possible connection between the emergence of nursing employment for women and women's exclusion from organised medicine. Clark suggests that progressive discrimination against female practitioners by medical craft guilds was symptomatic of a wider trend in the seventeenth century in which women were also prevented from entering the rising male professions of the law, military and some skilled trades. Clark attributed this to developing capitalist economic organisation which moved the locus of skilled work out of the family to the market where corporate organisations progressively dominated the provision of certain skills, such as healing, once carried on primarily by women in the family. Agencies of occupational control, such as the medical corporations, became *de facto* and subsequently *de jure* male preserves in a society in which women had few if any powers outside the increasingly limited purview of the family.

We would suggest that the formal exclusion of women from the male 'empirics' guilds, coupled with the development of hospitals, and a substantial middle class in the eighteenth century, meant favourable conditions for the extended employment of women as nurses in the public and private sphere. But even in the early eighteenth century, women were not necessarily pushed into nursing work, and healers were still often classified according to specific skills rather than sex, such as the women appointed to St Bartholomew's Hospital in 1708 to treat skin cases.[29]

It was in the nineteenth century that rigid distinctions were finally enforced between 'curing' and 'caring' functions, which were allocated to male doctors and female nurses respectively. A recent sociological study shows that the modern conception of the nurse's role was very much a product of nineteenth-century English society. It delineates how nursing reform drew various ideological supports from Victorian stereotypes of 'femininity'. The drunken old hag image of the nurse was refashioned by Nightingale and others into a respectable, angelic, obedient wife/mother symbol romanticised in the bourgeois family. Hence the passive role assigned to women in the nineteenth-century middle-class home lent symbolic weight to the subordinate place assigned to women in the health sphere. These ideas cast the doctor into an heroic mould as saviour of the sick, whilst the nurse was relegated to the mundane housekeeping chore of managing an hygienic environment for her patient and to the 'womanly' business of caring. The author shows that sexual divisions created in the family transplanted perfectly to the workplace. Nursing reformers' zeal created a home from home for the medical man in the sickroom where the nurse/wife provided practical and symbolic supports for the doctor akin to those found in his own drawing room.[30]

This type of approach opposes the historical convention of nursing as a 'naturally' feminine role by showing that the nurse's role, as we know it today, derives from an historically specific value system about sex roles. Those values prescribed how men and women were expected to behave in sick care at a particular point in time, but were neither, as historical orthodoxy has often implied, empirical descriptions of healing roles that had always obtained nor factual statements about the intrinsic 'natural' properties of men and women.

By now it is clear that a great deal of potential evidence exists about women's past which could enable us to construct a very different kind of history of health care. But it is also evident that we must begin that history with some new questions.

Towards an Alternative History of Women Healers

We could begin from very different premises from those that have informed most histories of health care. We can be explicitly critical of history which has been written solely from a male viewpoint, and propose instead that we should re-examine the past from the point of view of women. This differs from the kinds of histories we have criticised, in so far as our values are explicitly stated and women are given centre stage as the primary focus of analysis. Since there is a social power and status difference between the sexes, we can assume that male and female interests differ. Moreover, we can expect that differences of power and interest between men and women will be manifested in the health sector as in other spheres of social life. Indeed, health care can be seen not simply as a neutral site for the benevolent care of the sick, but also as an arena in which the sexes have historically competed over who should control and deliver healing services. Male attempts to dominate healing have generated a variety of ideologies devaluing women as healers, and one of our basic tasks should be to recognise this as ideology and treat it accordingly. Women's past skills as healers cannot be dismissed as mere old wives' tales, and we can insist upon a positive rather than a negative status for women in history. In contrast to conventional histories we can suggest that women healers have always played a crucial role in maintaining the health and physical well-being of the population. Furthermore, we should not forget that collective female healing effort in the past was often of relative therapeutic efficacy for the period, and usually provided a valuable social service to the poor, who otherwise had little chance of receiving care. Evidence cited earlier from the work of Hughes and Clark suggests that we would be on firm, if little-explored, historical territory. But, to date, the evidence is limited and fragmentary, and we need a great deal more. It will only become available if women's past healing work is treated as a topic worthy of serious investigation, and not dismissed or trivialised, as it has been in orthodox histories. Therefore we need to map out the terrain of women's healing functions in considerable detail.

We should ask many more detailed questions about which tasks were performed by whom, and for which patients. When were many healing functions once performed by women differentiated and sex-typed and for what reasons? To what extent did the sexual differentiation of many healing functions devolve from developments indigenous to sick care, from changing social attitudes to illness, or from other changes in the environing society? In which fields of work, social settings, markets, institutions and social classes were changes in the roles of personnel according to sex manifested? How did these occupational changes interact with or reflect social changes in the family, economy, the nature of work and social position of the sexes? Is Clark correct in positing a polarisation between the family and market-based corporate organisation of skill, as a key to female exclusion from medical practice? Questions of this type raise an ever widening circle of historical issues about the social management of health and illness, the internexus between health care practice and the social fabric, and the fluctuating position and roles of men and women. Further, the data which these questions could yield would permit us to address a central question as to how and why in the past women had lost control of healing to the male medical profession.

One imaginative and provocative attempt to address this question was offered by two feminists, Barbara Ehrenreich and Deidre English, in their short programmatic pamphlet, 'Witches, Midwives and Nurses: A History of Women Healers' (hereafter referred to as WMN), which first appeared in 1973.[31] The pamphlet rapidly became the token feminist statement in the field and gained considerable constituency in the women's movement, amongst health workers and those with an academic interest in the health sector. The argument is schematic and the pamphlet is quite deliberately written for a popular audience. Perhaps because of this, the piece has attracted little detailed critique from scholars and researchers. In what follows we shall attempt to provide such a critique, less to indict the pamphlet's weaknesses than as a way of advancing the authors' intentions by raising problems requiring research effort. Evidence from the English context is used, not to disprove the pamphlet, but rather to assess how far its ideas could contribute to a detailed investigation of women's past healing role in this country.

Although subtitled, somewhat misleadingly, 'A History of Women Healers', the pamphlet by no means pretends to provide a complete chronological account; instead it focuses on what it calls two distinct phases in the male medical 'take-over' of healing. One of these phases concerns medieval England and Europe, the other nineteenth-century America (the authors' domicile). This effectively divides the pamphlet into two main sections which we will deal with in order. The first section treating the medieval period contains some of WMN's most controversial arguments. Here the authors build on Hughes's point that peasant women healers were sometimes persecuted for witchcraft, and marry this with other studies about medieval witch persecution to claim that witchmania was central in what they regard as the destruction of female influence over healing by a nascent medical profession, male ruling class and church. The authors give most space to the fate of what they see as 'the great mass of female healers – the "witches" ', whom they claim were persecuted by the male establishment between the fourteenth and seventeenth centuries in the witchmania which swept across Europe and resulted in the execution of hundreds of thousands of women. WMN suggests that peasant healers were part of a rebellious underground social movement, the beliefs and subversive political potential of which threatened and opposed the authority of the church and male aristocracy. In addition, many women in this informal network were healers whose curative success also threatened doctors with whom these women competed for patients. Church, state and medical men are believed to have united to suppress these women, and accused them of black magic, sexual and spiritual congress with the devil, and the use of demonic powers to cure the sick.

WMN may be making a very inspired guess at some of the political connotations of witch hunts. Undoubtedly, the vast majority of witches were women, and witch hunts were a widespread European phenomenon between the fourteenth and seventeenth centuries. A medieval historian recently commented that 'misogyny takes many forms, but it has seldom provided a legal rationale for killing dozens of thousands of women (and a few men as well), such as that provided by the capital crime of witchcraft'.[32] Despite the verifiable misogyny of witchmania and its undoubted use against poor women, there are considerable difficulties in invoking the witchcraft argument as a general blanket explanation for loss of female influence over healing, particularly in English society, and we must see why. This is important since WMN's witchcraft thesis has provoked conflicting responses which usually leave us in an impasse. Non-specialists have often accepted the argument as basically correct and have therefore assumed that little additional research is required to validate it. At the other extreme, many historians have dismissed the pamphlet out of hand, as mere sensational feminist polemic. Somewhere between these two extremes, other readers have been inspired by the audacity of the argument, but have felt unable to extend it, or criticise it properly, without detailed knowledge of medieval history. Whichever stance has been adopted, the result has been stalemate. Witchmania is one of the great scholarly puzzles of history and debate has raged for more than a century over the origins, causes and implications of witch persecution. Without taking on that vast debate we can nevertheless enter it through examining the imputed connection between witchcraft and healing. This is fundamental to WMN's argument, but is also extremely contentious on empirical grounds.

In England we know that not all female healers were witches, let alone the mass of them, whilst recorded prosecutions for witchcraft in this country, whether these involved healers or not, and they mostly did not, were much less numerous than in Continental Europe.[33] Women are often cited in the witchcraft literature as causing illness, but are mentioned less often in a healing role, although midwifery was alleged to have had particular connections with demonology.[34] One critic claims that 'there is not the slightest evidence that many women tried as witches were actually lay healers, much less the great majority of them'.[35] WMN supports its witchcraft—healing thesis *inter alia* by the suggestion that, in an era of limited understanding of disease, female healers' curative success probably appeared magical and was thus attributed to the devil's influence. But Hughes shows that women's therapeutic success was also often attributed to saintliness, purity and a favoured relationship with the Almighty, and the canonisation of women devoted to the sick would tend to support this view. Further, a recent study of medieval images of women shows that medieval society subscribed to a dichotomous model of feminity, in which purity was imputed to the aristocratic woman who was put on a pedestal, in contrast to the evil imputed to the peasant woman who was often burnt at the stake or hanged.[36] The pedestal and the stake provided contradictory models of feminity, and the aristocratic lady might be revered as a saint of the sick, whilst the peasant wise woman could be seen as a dangerous and powerful witch. Hence, class is a crucial consideration, since women were not, nor are they now, an homogeneous group; thus any theory must take account of class differences between women.

The authors of WMN cite medical involvement in witch trials as evidence of medical attempts to outlaw competing women, but one critic claims that:

> physicians were used mainly as expert witnesses to help the court decide whether the alleged victims of witchcraft died or became ill from natural or supernatural causes, or whether any of the accused women had typical signs of being a witch . . . Often physicians testified against supernatural intervention (i.e. in favour of the accused) in fact one of the earliest and most outspoken defences of women accused of witchcraft came from John Weyer, an influential physician.[37]

The medical role in witch trials is thus at best ambiguous, and for this and other reasons, not least the possible relevance of the witchcraft argument only to peasant women, Ehrenreich and English's thesis about witchcraft may not be very useful for understanding women's loss of social status as healers.

Some critics of the pamphlet believe that WMN's entire thesis of competition between medical men and women collapses because women only served the poor, whilst medical men provided services to the 'court and clergy'.[38] In sum, the sexes are believed to have served 'different social classes'.[39] Yet this assumption is only possible because the existence of educated upper-class female healers has been ignored by critics; in fact, the authors of WMN themselves make only very

brief reference to women of the upper class, whom they claim were the
object of a successful outlawing campaign by the medical profession
'throughout Europe' by the fourteenth century. But Hughes and Clark
show that, although upper-class women ministered to the poor as
befitted 'persons of quality', these ladies also seem to have acted as
unofficial physicians and surgeons to other members of the aristocracy
and gentry, thus directly competing with elite gentlemen physicians and
lesser surgeons and apothecaries. Clark suggests that this situation
obtained until well into the seventeenth century and cites a number of
such women, e.g. Lady Falkland who was well known for 'providing
antidotes against infection and of Cordials, and other several sorts of
physick for such of her neighbours as should need them . . . her skil was
indeed more than ordinary and her wariness too'. A clergyman reports
that 'My L. Honeywood sent her coach for me; . . . my lady was my
nurse and Phisitian and I hope for much good'. Whilst Mrs Bedell 'was
very famous and expert in Chirurgery which she continually practised
upon multitudes that flock'd to her . . . without respect of persons poor
or rich'.[40] Indeed, if skilled educated women had not competed with
various categories of medical men, it is unlikely that the denigration of
female practice would constitute such a strong theme in past medical
writings, or that female healers in England and elsewhere would have
been prosecuted for what were seen as infringements on licensed
physicians' and surgeons' practices. If, as medical historians have
implied, female healers had been primarily religious mystics or illiterate
incompetent old wives, they would hardly have constituted any threat
to respectable medical practitioners.

Yet evidently women did constitute a threat. Aside from royal
edicts, the fragmented medical occupations made attempts to outlaw
female practice, although these were largely ineffectual because of the
difficulty of bringing sanctions to bear on offenders who would
probably have been defended by grateful patients anyway. Nevertheless,
the exclusion of women from the recognised practice of 'physick' by
the Royal College of Physicians, followed by progressive exclusion of
women from male 'empirics' guilds, undoubtedly created a primitive
sexual differentiation and division between men and women which
would pave the way for a rigid and formal sexual division of labour in
healing when medical men finally united in one profession in 1858. It
would seem that a thesis of competition between male doctors and
women could be a very fruitful line of inquiry and should be explored
and researched in detail. In fact, we lack any labour history of the
health sphere, especially from the point of view of women. (Cf.

Carpenter in this volume.) Such a history could contribute much to our understanding of the development of the health occupations and their respective statuses in the division of labour.

Given the brevity of WMN, it would be churlish to accuse the authors of omitting what they never intended to include. Nevertheless, having chosen a dual focus — i.e. on pre-seventeenth-century England and Europe, then nineteenth-century America — the authors offer no discernible bridge between the two periods or continents save two or three brief paragraphs referring to the seventeenth and eighteenth centuries in England. This is rather unfortunate since it could convey the erroneous impression that the principal eras of change in the position of women healers occurred before the seventeenth century, then during and after the nineteenth century, with little of note happening between them. However, the seventeenth and eighteenth centuries were extremely important periods of general social trans-formation in England and, although under-researched, a few studies of the period offer initial clues indicating ferment in the health field and probable fluctuations in the social position of women within it.

Thus, for example, one of the foremost social historians of seventeenth-century England, Christopher Hill, analyses conflicts between protagonists of popular and academic science and medicine, disputes between groups of healers, connections between socio-political, religious and scientific dissent, and revolutionary Puritan ideas about the social status of the sexes.[41] All of this has obvious relevance to the evolution of past healing practice and aspects of women's role within it. Other studies provide evidence of municipal regulation of healers' work (although the implications for women are not investi-gated), whilst the issue of collective organisation by groups of women is raised by the response of seventeenth-century midwives to male medical invasion of their field through unsuccessful attempts to achieve autonomous corporate secular organisation. In this period male medical guilds were beginning to formalise their own organisations to protect their interests, and we may well ask whether other groups of female healers, aside from midwives, also attempted to organise collectively to further their own occupational interests. Clark suggests that women were fairly widely employed by church and other authorities to nurse the sick poor, to tend people 'stricken with smallpox or the plague', to search bodies for causes of death, and to visit the infirm. Hence a considerable female network seems to have existed, performing important social and health care services about which we know little.

The eighteenth century was probably a very significant watershed in social management of health and illness, for an urban-based voluntary hospital system for the acutely sick poor grew up in this period. Also, there was a vast growth in the 'middling classes' of society, providing a new market for medical services and a rapid expansion of numbers of medical practitioners of all kinds who increasingly tried to close and professionalise their own occupations. By the end of the century the general practitioner had emerged, no doubt impinging on the extent of female involvement in health care amongst the middle and upper classes, whilst massive urbanisation and industrialisation at the end of the century must have had far-reaching consequences for health, sick care, family life and the ability of women in the family to cope with its health needs, especially in the working class where women joined the industrial labour force in large numbers.

The second half of WMN deals with the rise of the nineteenth-century American medical profession, the related suppression of popular and women's health movements, and the creation of American hospital nursing on the Nightingale model. This can be compared with the British experience. Much of the detailed information in this section shows the striking historical differences between the two societies. But we can draw out a few points of general interest. The American case is extreme, in so far as the male take-over of healing was much more extensive than in England, female midwifery disappeared completely in most states in the early decades of this century, and 100 per cent doctor delivery rapidly became the norm except in the most outlying rural areas. Female entry to the medical profession was curtailed even more severely than in England, and even today women constitute only 7 per cent of practising physicians. Indeed, it was clear that women were only to be allowed to work in the American health care system as 'a unified maid service' to male professionals, either as nurses or in other later paramedical occupations.

WMN rightly or wrongly implies a continuity between what occurred in Europe and later in the New World which is put at the extreme of a continuum in which women have been ousted from control of the health services. WMN insists that this is a political issue which has engaged other socially underprivileged groups such as working people and members of ethnic minority groups, who in the USA also fought a losing battle against a powerful male profession and upper class. The authors try to show that conflicts over who controls and delivers health care services cannot be understood in isolation from the rest of society, but rather mirror the ideas and aspirations of a variety of social and political movements. In the American case, groups that lost the battle were asking radical questions not just about the content of health services, but about their control by a small coterie of male professionals. This questions the distribution of power and privilege in society as a whole. It is an argument for an historical approach which would interpret changes in health occupations in relation to a wide range of social issues, especially the interests and actions of groups other than male professionals. This would imply a history of health care from 'below', rather than primarily from 'above' as in orthodox histories (see Carpenter in this volume). It would also draw attention to many neglected political aspects of the health care system, and especially to the way in which power differences between the sexes have permeated and shaped the health division of labour.

This chapter has tried to provide some new questions for the research that will have to be done to recapture our history as health workers. Indeed, there is a rich seam of questions and controversies that can be mined for research purposes, in order to begin an alternative history of health care. This alternative would inevitably formulate new hypotheses, not just about women but about the entire social environment of past sick care. It could only bring us closer to understanding the past 'as it really was', which is surely the purpose of history.

We should not forget that throughout the ages women have willingly cared for the helpless, infirm and socially dependent, but that the reward for this valuable social service has too often been indifference, scorn, or the status of a servant class. We do not know why this has happened with such consistency, nor why women's caring has been so devalued in our society, but perhaps history could provide some answers from the past and suggest an alternative for the future.

Notes

1. For example, R. Briedenthal and C. Koonz (eds), *Becoming Visible* (Houghton Mifflin, Boston, 1977); B. A. Carroll (ed.), *Liberating Women's History* (University of Illinois Press, Illinois, 1976); M. Hartman and L. W. Banner, *Clio's Consciousness Raised* (Harper and Row, London, 1974).

2. This is a generalisation, but applies to the vast majority of secondary sources in the history of medical ideas and institutions, health care occupations and social policies on health in so far as these refer or not to women's role in healing. A representative sample of this literature can be found in the Wellcome Library for the History of Medicine, Wellcome Institute, London. There are some exceptions to this trend which are not cited in this chapter: e.g. N. and J. Parry, *The Rise of the Medical Profession* (Croom Helm, London, 1976), Ch. 8, 'Sexual Divisions and the Medical Occupations'; J. Woodward and D. Richards (eds), *Health Care and Popular Medicine in Nineteenth Century England* (Croom Helm,

London, 1977), Chs 2, 3, 4; A. Mclaren, *Birth Control in Nineteenth Century England* (Croom Helm, London, 1978); L. Gordon, *Woman's Body, Woman's Right* (Grossman Publishers, New York, 1976). Secondly, there is a small but growing volume of studies which are explicitly critical of past medical ideas about and attitudes to women's bodies, personalities and diseases; amongst the best known are B. Ehrenreich and D. English, *Complaints and Disorders: The Sexual Politics of Sickness* (Glass Mountain Pamphlet no. 2, New York, 1974), and R. and J. Haller, *The Physician and Sexuality in Nineteenth Century America* (University of Illinois Press, Illinois, 1974).

3. See, for example: C. Hill, *Intellectual Origins of the English Revolution* (Panther Books, London, 1972), Ch. 2, especially pp. 74–84; B. M. Smith, 'Some Aspects of the Medical Profession in Eighteenth Century England, Considered as a Factor in the Rise of the Professional Middle Classes', unpublished PhD thesis, London, 1951; B. Hamilton, 'The Medical Profession in the Eighteenth Century', *Econ. Hist. Review*, vol. IV, no. 2 (1951); J. M. Peterson, *The Medical Profession in Mid-Victorian London* (University of California Press, London, 1978).

4. This is evident in the eighteenth- and nineteenth-century literature on childbirth management when medical men were trying to dominate midwifery practice, and the derogation of midwives' competence gave rise to extensive medical polemic.

5. H. Smith, 'Gynaecology and Ideology in Seventeenth Century England', in Carroll, *Liberating Women's History*.

6. A notable exception is C. Woodham-Smith, *Florence Nightingale* (Constable, London, 1950).

7. M. S. Newby, 'Florence Nightingale a Woman of All-Time: Myths and Stereotypes', in *Society for the Social History of Medicine Bulletin*, 18 (1976). This gives a succinct overview of the Nightingale literature.

8. E.g. the classic work by M. A. Nutting and L. Dock, *A History of Nursing* (Putnam, New York, 1907); B. and V. L. Bullough, *The Emergence of Modern Nursing* (Macmillan, New York, 1964); B. Abel-Smith, *A History of the Nursing Profession* (Heinemann, London, 1960).

9. R. White, *Social Change and the Development of the Nursing Profession* (Henry Kimpton, London, 1978).

10. Although medical men first began midwifery practice in England in the late seventeenth century, the profession did not recognise midwifery as a legitimate branch of medicine until the second Medical Registration Act of 1886, when proficiency in midwifery became a formal prerequisite of basic medical registration.

11. J. Donnison, *Midwives and Medical Men: A History of Inter-Professional Rivalries and Women's Rights* (Heinemann, London, 1977).

12. J. H. Aveling, *English Midwives: Their History and Prospects* (1872) (reprint, Hugh K. Elliott Ltd, London, 1967).

13. A very recent exception is R. W. and D. C. Wertz, *Lying-In: A History of Childbirth in America* (Schocken Books, New York, 1979).

14. Cited by E. Gamarnikow, 'Sexual Division of Labour: the case of Nursing', in A. Kuhn and A. M. Wolpe, *Feminism and Materialism* (Routledge and Kegan Paul, London, 1978), p. 115.

15. Ibid., p. 105.

16. M. Simms, 'The Woman Hater', *Spare Rib*, no. 85. See also M. Simms, 'The Medical Woman Question', *World Medicine*, vol. 14, no. 10 (1979); E. Blackwell, *Pioneer Work in Opening the Medical Profession to Women* (1912) (reprint, Schocken Books, New York, 1977), Ch. 9; R. Strachey, *The Cause* (1928) (reprint, Virago Books, London, 1978).

17. Gamarnikow, 'Sexual Division of Labour', pp. 98–101.

18. S. Jex Blake, *Medical Women: A Thesis and A History* (Hamilton, Adams and Co., London, 1886).

19. A. Clark, *Working Life of Women in the Seventeenth Century* (George Routledge and Sons, London, 1919); E. Power, 'Women Practitioners of Medicine in the Middle Ages', *Proc. Royal Society of Medicine* (1921); K. C. Hurd-Mead, *A History of Women in Medicine from the Earliest Times to the Beginning of the Nineteenth Century* (Haddam Press, Haddam, Conn., 1938); M. J. Hughes, *Woman Healers in Medieval Life and Literature* (Morningside Heights, New York, 1943).

20. S. Chaff *et al.*, *Women in Medicine: A Bibliography of Literature on Women Physicians* (Scarecrow Press, Inc., Metuchen, New Jersey and London, 1977).

21. Power, 'Women Practitioners', pp. 21, 23.

22. Clark, *Working Life*, p. 255.

23. G. Clark, *A History of the Royal College of Physicians of London* (Clarendon Press, Oxford, 1964), pp. 132, 188, 517.

24. Smith, *Some Aspects of the Medical Profession*; Hamilton, 'The Medical Profession'.

25. *Select Committee on Medical Registration* (London, 1847); S. W. F. Holloway, 'Medical Education in England 1830–1858', *History*, 49 (1964); and Peterson, *The Medical Profession*.

26. See Strachey, *The Cause*.

27. Clark, *Working Life*, p. 258.

28. Ibid., pp. 257, 258.

29. The last such appointment was made in 1708: N. Moore, *History of St. Bartholomew's Hospital*, vol. II (Pearson, London, 1918), p. 733. The hospital archives contain a great deal of material on women's medical work in the hospital, including records of payments to women brought into the hospital to exercise special skills or effect particular cures.

30. Gamarnikow, 'Sexual Division of Labour'.

31. Reprinted in England by the Writers and Readers Publishing Co-operative (1977).

32. W. E. Monter, 'The Pedestal and the Stake: Courtly Love and Witchcraft', in R. Briedenthal and C. Koonz (eds), *Becoming Visible*, p. 133.

33. Ibid.

34. See A. Oakley, 'Changes in the Management of Childbirth', in A. Oakley and J. Mitchell (eds), *The Rights and Wrongs of Women* (Penguin Books, Harmondsworth, 1976).

35. V. V. and D. Ozonoff, 'Steps Towards a Radical Analysis of Health Care', *International Journal of Health Services*, vol. 5 (1975), pp. 299–303.

36. Monter, 'The Pedestal'.

37. Ozonoff, 'Steps Towards a Radical Analysis'.

38. Ibid.

39. L. Doyal, S. Rowbotham and A. Scott, Introduction to English edition of *Witches, Midwives and Nurses: A History of Women Healers* (Writers and Readers Publishing Co-operative, London, 1977), p. 12.

40. Clark, *Working Life*, pp. 256–7.

41. See Hill, *Intellectual Origins*, and C. Hill, *The World Turned Upside Down* (Penguin Books, London, 1975).

9 ARCHIVES AND THE HISTORY OF NURSING

Janet Foster and Julia Sheppard

Whether a researcher uses primary sources, secondary sources or, as is usual, a mixture of both is dictated by the state of knowledge in the area, the way the problem has been formulated, time available and so on. A crucial factor in all this is the degree of familiarity the researcher has with potential sources and ways of seeking them out. Janet Foster and Julia Sheppard are both experienced archivists who have responsibilities for and an interest in records in the field of health. Their discussion brings home the crucial importance of background knowledge as a prelude to the search for historical records. These writers are familiar with the relevant government bodies, the charitable associations and so on. They couple this with their specialist knowledge of the likely location of records of various sorts and with information about key reference publications. A great deal of useful information is packed into a short space here and it should serve to widen our horizons. Finding a completely new source can be exhilarating, of course, but working with different sources from the conventional ones and asking new questions of old sources can be just as rewarding. Archivists can help us to consider new options but, in the end, it is the researcher who must make the choice, the researcher who must formulate the questions and marshal the data.

————Ed.

The strict definition of an archive is a document which is produced by an individual or institution in the normal course of life or work and which provides a record or part of the history of that individual or institution. Archives are mainly written documents — that is, manuscript or typescript — but photographs and sound recordings can also be classified as archives, as can some printed material. For example, the printed annual reports of a hospital form part of its archives and, as such, would be considered a primary source, whereas a published history of a hospital is a secondary source. In this article we are not concerned exclusively with manuscript sources but with a whole range of different information-recording materials.

A basic problem with studying the history of nursing is that before c. 1860 there is very little direct documentary evidence. It was not until after the revolution in nursing, begun by Florence Nightingale and continued by Mrs Bedford Fenwick, that there were professionals who created their own records. It was not until the establishment of schools of nursing, which embodied the new approach to nursing, that any nursing administration records began to be kept. From then on we may expect to find matron's weekly and annual reports, registers of probationers and students, and even student nurses' notebooks, all of which may be termed direct archives. However, the increased interest in nursing at this period led to the subject being dealt with in a variety of other, less obvious, records, and this diversity of sources is one of the main problems when approaching research into any aspect of the history of nursing. It is, therefore, the aim of this chapter to discuss the sources available, the type of information they may be expected to contain, their location and means of access to them, as well as to discuss, briefly, how to use archives for research purposes.

We have stated that there are, strictly speaking, no nursing archives before there were nursing professionals who created their own records; nevertheless, from the medieval period onwards, there are records through which we may obliquely approach the history of nurses. Although it is true that the modern nurse cannot trace her ancestry in a direct line from the sisters in the medieval religious houses, a chronological survey of sources for the history of nursing must begin with the records of these medieval sisters. One such, for example, was Isabel, daughter of Edward de Bray, who gave her house to the monks of St Bartholomew's Hospital early in the twelfth century so that she might enter the community and perform the duties of a sister in caring for the sick poor. The charter recording Isabel's gift, and the reason for it, is preserved in the archives of St Bartholomew's[1] and it is to be expected that similar documents survive in the records of other hospitals that were founded in the Middle Ages. Unfortunately, no records survive of the village women, of that time and of later, who attended childbed and prepared herbal remedies, often receiving payment in kind, occasionally being hounded as witches.

After the Reformation, when religious institutions were suppressed by Henry VIII covetous of their lands and treasures, the hospitals that survived did so as voluntary, lay organisations run by unpaid Boards of Governors. It is the minutes of the meetings of these Boards of Governors that provide the single most informative source for institutional nursing from the mid-sixteenth to the eighteenth century. During this period all matters concerning the running of a hospital came before the governors, or a select committee of them, for discussion. Again, St Bartholomew's provides an example: the very first recorded meeting of the governors of the hospital in 1549 ordered the provision of russet cloth for the matron's livery or uniform, whilst an order of 1554, that lengths of watchett, a blue cloth, should be purchased for

the sisters' liveries, establishes the antiquity of blue uniforms.[2] Details
of the duties of the nursing staff may be gathered from minutes which
will reflect the developing hierarchy within a hospital and the changing
role of the sisters.[3] Other details of remuneration, pensions, allowances
of food and ale will appear, incidentally, in hospital minutes, whilst
treasurers' accounts contain a full record of salaries and payments.
These are the documents and the type of information they may yield
about women who worked in hospitals between 1540 and 1800. Such
records, of course, continue into the following centuries but become
less important with the growth of other, more direct, sources.

Nothing has been said so far about nurses other than those working
in hospitals. This is because records of nursing outside regular
institutions before the nineteenth century are scarce, to say the least.
Usually the sick who were not poor would be nursed in their own
homes by relatives, advised by a physician whose services would be
paid for. Here it is sometimes possible to find references amongst
collections of family papers, perhaps in a diary or among bills and
receipts, to a nurse being employed, although such research is likely to
involve a great deal of work for little return. More easily accessible
information comes from biographies and novels. However, these latter
must be used with caution. Were there really such tyrants as Grace
Poole who watched over the unfortunate Mrs Rochester in *Jane Eyre*?
It was characters such as that which created the popular image of
nurses as gin-swilling harridans and contributed to the revolution in
nursing witnessed during the nineteenth century, but we must beware
of accepting these popular images, and the more polemical reports of
the reformers, without question.

When we reach the nineteenth century, the sources become more
plentiful and varied. Some independent training schools predated
hospital-attached schools and it is worth bearing in mind that, if these
later amalgamated with a hospital, the records should have been
transferred.[4] With the establishment of schools of nursing, registers of
probationers and students begin, giving details of their progress
through training and, often, of their subsequent careers or otherwise.
One of the first probationers at St Bartholomew's in 1877 was
dismissed after three months for 'indiscreet and light conduct with
Patients'.[5] Lecture notebooks form another source: those of the more
industrious students may survive, giving some indication of the content
and scope of courses, something which would also be reflected in
surviving examination papers. Then there are the matron's report books
and the range of records attendant upon the growth of nursing

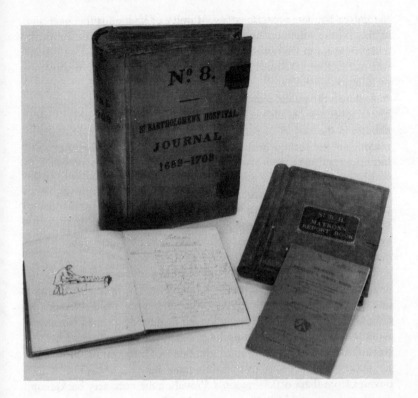

administration as a separate entity. However, this is all still concentrating on the voluntary hospitals, whereas the nineteenth century saw a vast increase in the numbers of destitute patients attended to in the infirmaries that developed as part of the workhouse system under the jurisdiction of the parish poor law Boards of Governors. As nursing moved into the public sector, much wider and more varied source material becomes available. With increased public concern there were debates in the Houses of Parliament, select committees gathering evidence in the form of verbal depositions by nurses, parliamentary inquiries resulting in reports on workhouse infirmary conditions, all of which can be found among the records of Parliament. And, of course, parliamentary archives become essential during the period of Mrs Bedford Fenwick's campaign for state registration which produced select committees in 1904 and 1905, with their wealth of verbatim evidence, as well as the Acts of Parliament[6] and attendant debates both in and out of the House.

By the turn of the century a number of societies concerning nursing had been established the records of which reflect work in hospitals and outside them. Minute books, accounts, annual reports and correspondence of, for example, the Association for Promoting Trained Nursing in Workhouse Infirmaries, the Hospitals' Association and the British Nurses' Association should yield a great deal of information, although the reasons for the decisions that were made may not always be obvious from these official records. Providing the necessary background details is one aspect of the importance of private papers. These may include letters, diaries, memoranda, lecture notes or memoirs, where may be found a rough note or comment about a personality or a situation that can explain pages of official policy. In relation to nursing history, personal observations, rather than the solely administrative records, may give particularly vital evidence.

To turn to printed sources, *The Times* provides one of the best records of social change and shifts in public opinion. The background to and progress of the reform in nursing may be followed in newspapers and journals, which often influenced the creation of official records. An instance of this is afforded by the events following the death of one Timothy Daly in Holborn Workhouse in 1864 from 'filthiness caused by gross neglect'.[7] The incident was taken up by the press and *The Lancet* commissioned three doctors to visit all the London workhouse infirmaries and report on them. These reports were systematically published by *The Lancet* and led to an official parliamentary inquiry and report culminating in the Metropolitan Poor Act of 1867. Florence

Nightingale was reportedly 'so much obliged to that poor man for dying' — a sentiment that may be heartily endorsed by the student of nursing history surveying the plethora of records to which his death ultimately gave rise.

Among printed sources, journals in general must also be considered, and in the nineteenth century they abounded. There are the obvious: *Nursing Record*, later the *British Journal of Nursing*; the *British Medical Journal*, which in 1894 began its own series of Special Commission Reports on the Nursing and Administration of Provincial Workhouses; and *Hospital*. Apart from these, there are the less likely sources such as the *St. Paul's Monthly Magazine* and the *Cornhill Magazine* which regularly had articles about all aspects of medical care, and also *Burdett's Hospital and Annual Yearbook* which gives a yearly account of the progress in nursing as well as quantities of useful statistics. Last but not least should be mentioned the journals produced by the hospitals themselves, which often include first-hand accounts of life on the wards, helping to flesh out the rather dry bones of official reports. For example, a poetic portrayal of New Year's Eve in the Edinburgh Infirmary in 1873 begins:

Kate the scrubber (forty summers
stout but sportive) treads a measure

and continues to describe the patients joining in the merriment:

Stumps are shaking, crutch-supported
Splinted fingers tap the rhythym[8]

The nineteenth century produced another dimension to archives — the visual record of photographs. Perhaps the most immediate conveyor of the 'feeling' of a period, a photograph can often tell more in a single image than can many pages of a written record. For instance, a photograph of a ward in the 1890s will show the nurses' uniforms of the time, the decoration and arrangement of the ward, which is the nurses' working environment, the equipment used and the types of patient being treated. This century too has contributed a new type of potential archive material in the form of sound and even video recording which may capture an entire occasion and preserve it for posterity. Recording can also be very useful when used deliberately, for example in taped interviews with people who would probably not commit their experiences and memories to writing; however, these must be treated with caution since they are conscious, and therefore subjective, records which may not give an unbiased account.

Where, then, may all these documents and records be found and what are likely to be the conditions attached to their access? Under the provisions of the Public Records Act of 1958, records of the National Health Service authorities, other than local health authorities, and of the National Health Service hospitals, with minor exceptions, are public records. This means that most hospital records are subject to the provisions of the Act, even though very few of the records are actually housed at the Public Records Office. The PRO does have some hospital records, for example those of the Elizabeth Garrett Anderson Hospital and, of course, the records of the Ministry of Health and its predecessors.[9] Generally speaking, access is allowed after 30 years to administrative records and after 100 years to medical records of patients. An important proviso to this is that the organisation concerned, which will normally mean the hospital administrators, may use its discretion in allowing access to records before this date, providing that individuals are not identified in any book or paper arising from the research undertaken.[10]

Sometimes hospital records may have been deposited at a local county or city record office, since NHS hospital records are regarded as a category of public record suitable for local deposit. It should be remembered that, since health records are only one of the many interests of a local archivist, he or she is not strictly under any legal obligation to house or locate them (although a certain moral obligation is present). Moreover, storage space and funding of local archives is frequently inadequate and the amount of time and energy that can be dedicated to hospital records will vary considerably from place to place.

In most cases the hospital will have kept its own records, unfortunately all too often unlisted and in poor storage conditions that will hasten the physical deterioration of the records. It is quite common that the hospital itself will not know what records exist or where they are housed. Only two hospitals in England have their own professional qualified archivists: St Bartholomew's Hospital and The Bethlem Royal and Maudsley Hospital. Some hospitals have 'honorary archivists' who are often retired doctors or consultants with an interest in the history of the hospital. In some cases these archivists or librarians have done invaluable work locating the records of the hospital or even retrieving them from offices and rubbish bins. Departments may be loath to give up their records, so that sometimes there will be large gaps in the papers that have been saved. At times of administrative changes, such as in 1948, much will have been discarded and, with the present closure of many NHS hospitals, it is feared that there may be many other records destroyed during the current financial crisis.

It is worth bearing in mind that libraries connected to hospitals or medical teaching schools may also have acquired or been offered papers and records considered to be of historical value, such as the correspondence or notes of an eminent physician attached to the hospital. The Barnes Medical Library at Birmingham is an example of this. Similarly, county record offices accept gifts or deposits and archives which may range from the minute books of a local benevolent society to a collection of papers of a local family. The emphasis here will, of course, be of local interest, but it is surprising what unexpected and interesting material can be found in local record offices. The county record office[11] will also house its own administrative records, which will include a range of local health care records from the 1834 Poor Law to present-day health visiting.[12] The records of institutions, associations and societies, if they are still active, will quite possibly be retained by them, or alternatively be deposited with a recognised repository. The Royal Colleges, for example, as well as many other groups not already mentioned, will probably have kept their own administrative records and correspondence. Bodies like the Royal College of Nursing are aware of the importance of saving historical archives, but in face of the usual problems of shortage of staff and space are unable to do a great deal even with their own non-current records.

The papers of founding or influential members of societies may be included with their archives. For example, the papers of Elizabeth Fry are kept in the Archives Department at the Friends' House in London. Collections of papers of well-known figures may well have found their way into national collections such as those at the British Library and the Bodleian Library in Oxford. Single or individual letters are sometimes placed in an 'Autograph Letter' category in libraries. The private papers of lesser-known personalities may be found literally anywhere, mouldering in attics or cellars, awaiting discovery by the zealous researcher. Photographs may be found in collections of papers or may form a complete collection on their own. The *Directory of British Photographic Collections* lists major collections in this country and has a good subject and personal name index. As mentioned above, oral history is a recent and growing field and some record offices are developing collections: radio and television programmes are selectively kept by the BBC Sound Archives.

Apart from local and national repositories, there are the specialist libraries and repositories of universities or institutions. The Wellcome Institute for the History of Medicine houses a unique library of the history of medicine with large Oriental manuscript, Western manuscript and autograph letter collections as well as the newly founded Contemporary Medical Archives Centre.[13] The School of Oriental and African Studies houses the papers of medical missionaries and nursing staff in India, Africa and China dating back to 1800. The British Library of Political and Economic Science (in the London School of Economics) has the records of the National Society of Children's Nurseries. The India Office houses the records of the Indian Nursing Service and government and missionary medical service records. The Department of Documents at the Imperial War Museum has documents relating to wartime nursing. Parliamentary papers, that is the records of Committees of Inquiry and Acts of Parliament, will be found amongst the records of Parliament in the House of Lords Record Office. Then there is the BBC Written Archives Centre which has the records of programmes made since 1922 and thus reflects the many different approaches to almost every subject in modern social and political history.

Newspapers usually maintain a complete set of back copies. *The Times* has its own established Archives Department, but in general the obvious place to consult is the British Library Newspaper Library at Colindale. The British Library can also be used for tracing articles in journals, but this is expected to be used as a last resort. Consult the British Union Catalogue of Periodicals (BUCOP) and see if it is possible to obtain the journal through your library or through inter-library loans.

Locating all these papers and records is not always easy and it is probably fair to say that the more original material that is sought, the more delving, letter writing and travelling the researcher is likely to have to undertake. There are, however, some obvious reference books and places that can be checked. One of the first places to consult is the National Register of Archives which acts under the aegis of the Royal Commission on Historical Manuscripts and which keeps a register of documents and collections known to be in recognised repositories and in private hands. It produces an *Annual List of Accessions to Repositories* based on information submitted by them. One of the drawbacks of the list is that it relies on information being submitted to it by a limited number of record repositories and the additional problem of the NRA index is that specialised subjects such as nursing do not appear in the subject index: the subject would have to be approached through classes of records such as those for associations or charities. Moreover, the personal name index is limited to those whose status is such that they have been included in the Dictionary of National Biography or equivalent; hence Florence Nightingale will appear, but not many other nurses. The NRA does hold copies of some lists of hospital records, as indeed does the PRO.

It is intended that the Contemporary Medical Archives Centre recently set up at the Wellcome Institute for the History of Medicine will be able to help researchers in this field, at least for the twentieth-century period. Apart from locating, cataloguing and, where relevant, receiving health and medical records and archives dating from 1900, the Centre also aims to build up a register of information on the whereabouts of such records. In the case of hospitals it is concentrating initially on all hospital records in London and the south east. To some extent the Centre will depend, like the National Register of Archives, on others supplying information to it, but it will also do a certain amount of field-work and make outline lists of relevant collections housed elsewhere.

Another obvious place to try is the local county or city record office or local history library. Record offices sometimes produce published guides and have lists and indexes of their accessions. It may well be worth while consulting the local archivist or librarian who may know of uncatalogued collections in their holdings or alternatively of the existence of relevant material held by local institutions. Archivists sometimes like to be informed about such material if they are unaware of it, for the record office might consider approaching the institution or individual directly for further information.

Finally, there is, of course, the direct approach by the historian or researcher. If you cannot find the information you require in any other way then it may be necessary to write yourself to the individual, society, hospital or association that you think may be able to help you. Assuming the body you wish to approach is still extant, a number of 'ifs' will govern your chances of success: if all the papers have been kept, if not, if it is known where they have gone, and if at the end of all this you are allowed access anyway.

This brings us to the somewhat thorny problem of access. It is essential to remember that (a) the material you wish to consult was not created with you, the historian, in mind but, on the whole, for purely administrative or personal reasons, (b) the archivist's primary responsibility is to safeguard the records, and (c) the archivist is neither historian nor librarian and you will be expected to do your own research on the records. With the exception of public records open under the 30-year rule, there is no divine right of access, and permission is at the discretion of the owner or legal representative. Conditions may be imposed which will appear unnecessarily harsh, or alternatively access will be given with surprisingly little restriction. In some cases it will be necessary to obtain a reader's ticket or sign an undertaking. Circumstances will affect this and, in spite of rumours to the contrary, archivists will try to help readers as much as possible, especially if such help is sought rather than demanded! In some cases archivists may prove an invaluable liaison between owner and historian, but they are bound by restrictions imposed by donors, depositors, the Public Record and Copyright Acts and their own judgement as to the dangers of allowing archives to be consulted. Since the first concern of the archivist is for the records, then he or she may feel obliged to withhold access if these are uncatalogued or in a poor condition or where their use would be unsupervised. It is usually better in the first instance to write explaining the research you intend to undertake and to enquire about conditions of access, the need for a reader's ticket, references, etc. It is then advisable to make an appointment to consult the archives, as this allows time for the relevant documents to be located and produced.[14] It should also be appreciated that the archivist does not exist to extract the information from the records and is not necessarily an authority on all they contain, but is primarily a custodian who will do his or her best to direct the researcher and to produce the records required. If research needs to be undertaken on the records and this cannot be done by the reader in person, a fee may be charged or the services of a professional researcher recommended.

Perhaps the most important point for all those wishing to use primary source material relating to nursing or any other subject is that the reader should approach the material with an open mind in order to get the most from it. Background reading is essential to put the particular area of subject in perspective and to learn which aspects have not been covered by published works and other generally available material. Having read around the subject, the next step is to see what the documents tell you rather than to look for individual theories to be proved. You may be surprised by your own conclusions.

Notes

1. St Bartholomew's Hospital Archives ref. Hcl/38.
2. SBH Archives ref. Hal/1 f. 1; f. 99v.
3. For example, the St Bartholomew's Hospital 'helpers', also called nurses,

were introduced into the wards in the seventeenth century, normally to take over
the more menial tasks such as 'beating the Bucke', which was an expression for
'doing the wash'; thereafter no sisters were appointed who had not had
experience as 'helpers'.

4. An example is the St John's House, founded in 1848, 'for the training and
employment of nurses for hospitals, the poor and private families'. It was finally
amalgamated with St Thomas' Hospital in 1920 and its records are at the Greater
London Record Office.

5. SBH Archives ref. MO11/4 p. 1. See also Ch. 2 where C. Maggs discusses
similar records in four provincial hospitals.

6. Nurses' Registration Act (1919), Nurses' Act (1943, 1949).

7. B. Abel-Smith, *A History of the Nursing Profession* (Heinemann, London,
1960), p. 42.

8. Quoted in full, ibid., p. 35.

9. Public Record Office, *Current Guide*. Ministry of Health (MH) Class
descriptions. Unpublished but available in the Search Room at the Public Record
Office.

10. For details of classes of hospital records which should be kept, see HM
(61)73, a circular entitled 'National Health Service: Preservation and Destruction
of Hospital Records'.

11. Every county in England and Wales, except Powys, has its own record
office. For London there is the Greater London Record Office at County Hall,
whilst many borough libraries also maintain archives.

12. It has been pointed out that nursing associations frequently made
contractual arrangements with the local authorities when the latter took over
district nursing services. Records arising from this may also be located at the
county records office. See J. Pickstone, 'Yes, but what was it *really* like?',
Journal of Community Nursing, March, 1980.

13. Sir Henry Wellcome (1853–1936) collected a vast amount of books and
manuscripts and these are the property of the Wellcome Trustees under the terms
of his will.

14. A useful discussion of this is provided by Ottley in a chapter entitled
'Access to Libraries and Archives: a Word to Users of this Guide on the Outside
Enquiry Problem'. This is to be found in G. Ottley, *Railway History: a guide to
Sixty-One Collections in Libraries and archives in Great Britain* (Library Associa-
tion, Subject Guide to Library Resources, no. 1, London, 1973), pp. 13–14.

Appendix 1: Reference Books and Background Reading

Accessions to Repositories and Reports added annually to the *National
Register of Archives* (HMSO, published annually).

Sectional List 17. Publications of the Royal Commission of Historical
Manuscripts (their published Reports and Calendars cover material up
to 1800 only).

Record Repositories in Great Britain (HMSO, 5th edn). (Details of
national local and institutional record offices. Unfortunately not as
detailed as the 4th edition.)

Directory of British Photographic Collections, compiled by John Wall (Royal Photographic Society Publication, Heinemann, London, 1977).

Archives and Local History, by F. G. Emmison (Methuen, 1966) (a practical guide to the discovery and use of local records, including some helpful books and journals).

The following are useful for their discussion of the types and uses of medical records:

Medical Records. An article by Charles Newman in *Archives, the Journal of the British Records Association*, vol. 1, no. 21 (1959).

Hospital Records. An article by N. J. M. Kerling in the *Journal of the Society of Archivists*, vol. V, no. 3 (1975), pp. 181–3.

Hospital Archives. An article by Patricia Allderidge in *British Hospital Journal and Social Services Review* (27 September 1968).

The Preservation of Medical and Public Health Records. Research Publication no. 1, produced by the Wellcome Unit for the History of Medicine, Oxford (1979).

Appendix 2: Useful Addresses

Archives Dept,
The Bethlem Royal Hospital and the Maudsley Hospital,
Monks Orchard Road,
Beckenham BR3 3BX

BBC Written Archives Centre,
Caversham Park,
Reading RG4 8TZ

British Library Newspaper Library,
Colindale Avenue,
London NW9 5HE

British Library of Political and Economic Science,
Houghton Street,
Aldwych,
London WC2A 2AE

House of Lords Records Office,
House of Lords,
London SW1A 0AA

Imperial War Museum,
Department of Libraries and Archives,
Lambeth Road,
London SE1 6HZ

India Office Library,
European Manuscripts Section,
Foreign and Commonwealth Office,
197 Blackfriars Road,
London SE1 8NG

National Register of Archives,
Quality House,
Quality Court,
Chancery Lane,
London WC2 1HP

Public Record Office,
Ruskin Avenue,
Kew,
Richmond,
Surrey TW9 4DU

Royal College of Nursing,
1 Henrietta Place,
London W1M 0AB

School of Oriental and African Studies Library,
Malet Street,
London WC1E 7HP

District Archives,
St Bartholomew's Hospital,
Smithfield,
London EC1A 7BE

Contemporary Medical Archives Centre,
The Wellcome Institute for the History of Medicine,
183 Euston Road,
London NW1 2BP

10 EPILOGUE

Charlotte Kratz

Writing an epilogue for this book is for me an exacting as well as an exciting experience. The reasons for my excitement will become evident, but it is for me an exacting task for I belonged for years to that group of persons who found history unutterably dull. At school it was certainly not my *forte*. Like many potential nurses I was a realist and could not be bothered with anything that seemed to have little relevance to what was going on around me — to the here and now. Geography, biology, foreign languages, even mathematics, these were things which one needed, which would help one to tackle both immediate and future problems. But history was dead and past, and time given to its mastery was time wasted in attaining mastery over life. Yet somewhere in my memory lurks a recollection of a single page in the otherwise stultifying dirge of a Roman history textbook — a page which seemed to address itself to my personal distant past and which therefore took on relevance and became vividly alive for me. Even during the time of the Roman Empire my forebears had struggled — and survived. I knew the page by heart and surprised both myself and my teacher by my sudden enthusiasm for history, alas short-lived. The next page was as dry and irrelevant again to my way of thinking as were its predecessors.

This brief experience in my youth of history as revelation, as illumination and more importantly as possible prediction, which has stayed with me for all this time, can now almost be seen as a premonition in its own right. For I have come to history over the years, not because I have mellowed and can now tolerate useless things, nor even because I like a good yarn (and much of real-life history is indeed stranger than the strangest fiction) but because I found in history those facts that help me to make the present intelligible through indicating the thought processes, the cultural and social mores, the legal and economic constraints, the human foibles and weaknesses and the chance events which caused history to take the particular turn it took at a particular moment.

But historical facts do more than that. Through illuminating those factors which led up to the present they help to indicate possible ways of shaping the future. Some forces which helped to shape our past are just as potent now as they were hundreds of years ago. The more intrepid may wish to meet them head on, to change society as it were, but those with more limited ambitions will simply wish to take them into account in their planning and, if possible, circumnavigate them. In the same way, the study of history will show us where social pressures, which are now irrelevant, influenced the present situation and where future plans should take into account the genesis of these factors so as to apply appropriate therapy for the healing of old wounds and subsequent healthy growth.

Of course, really to *use* history you need more than the sort of history on which many of us were brought up, the sort of history which after a cursory look at the monasteries moves straight on to the life of Florence Nightingale (and which was epitomised for me at a flower show devoted to the life of the saints and including among its exhibits one dedicated to Miss Nightingale). For nursing, the story of a saintly Victorian gentlewoman, chosen by the Almighty to 'create' nursing as we know it, has for nearly a century been wellnigh disastrous. Too many nurses have felt that this creation was immutable, and moreover that it had come about largely through ladylike submission to doctors and politicians alike.

Nothing could be further from the truth. Miss Nightingale was not only a prodigious worker, but her strategy of being an invalid probably not only helped her vast output of correspondence but also obliged men of influence to listen to her because of her invalidity in a way in which they might not otherwise have done. Yet even progress as spectacular as that set in motion by Miss Nightingale can only rarely occur as an isolated event, going against the stream of the times. The movement towards attracting respectable women to nursing only begins to make sense when it is set within the framework of what is rather inelegantly called 'the female surplus', the prevailing work ethic (only those who work shall eat — unless they are married women) and the demand by women not to be left out of the movement towards universal self-improvement. Furthermore, as Katherine Williams quite rightly reminds us, Miss Nightingale was not the first Englishwoman to proceed to Kaiserswerth — she had been preceded there by Elizabeth Fry. That Miss Nightingale (as well as Mr Rathbone of district nursing fame) found nurses with at least some preparation should alert us to the fact that not every nurse, even in the middle of the nineteenth century, was akin to 'Sarah Gamp'.

If there is one merit this book can claim above all others it is that it has not taken anything for granted. For those who, like me, are used to thinking of history as a collection of facts made dull by their very immutability, this may come as a surprise, if not as a shock. I am not implying that history is not a factual account of events as they actually happened, nor that the authors of this book ignore the facts. On the contrary, most of the authors have as their ultimate aim to confront us with facts of which we were not aware before, not because we were ignorant but because the questions had either never been asked or, having been asked, nobody had bothered to find answers.

Look, for example, at the chapter by Margaret Connor Versluysen. Why has the role of women as healers in their own right been neglected by historians? Why have attempts by women to help their fellow beings so often been ridiculed over the years and denigrated as witchcraft? Surely results, however achieved, should have commended recognition, particularly in an era which was not as blinkered to all but scientifically demonstrable truth as is ours? We are getting closer, today, to accepting the possibility of extra-sensory perception, of using non-scientific healing approaches like laying on of hands, hypnosis or acupuncture, but is it possible that this acceptance is predicated by its wider acceptability by men, convinced at last by the obvious inadequacies of the scientific method? Have we deprived humanity for years of means of improving its lot because such improvement would have come at the hands of women? And is this threat to progress in healing through the agency of women a thing of the past? Taking a feminist stance helps us not only to ask questions which have never been asked before but also to get an indication that the answers to such questions have considerable relevance for the present.

Mick Carpenter gives us another example of questions about nursing which have not been asked before, partly again because of sexually and morally based preconceptions — regarding nurses as equivalent to saintly women — but also because too often nursing is seen as a unitary profession instead of the conglomerate of divergent occupations it is in reality. Future historians may well wish to address themselves to the problem of why physiotherapists, social workers and dietitians have become known as professionals in their own right, while persons caring for the acutely physically sick in hospital, for the mentally ill and handicapped, for the long-term chronic sick, particularly those in their own homes, and for those mainly concerned with prevention have continued to be referred to collectively as nurses. By far the greatest interest in a history of nursing has centred on nursing the physically ill. Those nurses concerned with looking after the mentally ill seem to have taken on at least some of the stigma attached to those in their charge, in that few, if any, have looked at the history of the mental nurse and her, or more often his, predecessor — the asylum nurse. If we wish to consider this group of people as nurses in their own right, and they now constitute about 15 per cent of the collectivity of nurses and look after more than 50 per cent of those occupying hospital beds, then the least we can do is to acquaint ourselves with their antecedents. However, and more constructively, knowing their past should help us to understand their present position and perhaps enable us to use it in shaping our collective future.

I write this last sentence with some feeling, for, if there is one chapter I personally miss in this collection of accounts of our diverse pasts, it is an account of the development of the two major prongs of non-institutional nursing services — district nursing and health visiting. True, Dean and Bolton go some way in their analysis of the relationship between epidemics and district nursing to redress the balance, and many people will be aware that the Liverpool district nursing service did indeed become increasingly known and accepted following an outbreak of cholera in that town. But it is the difference in their upbringing — district nursing in the manor and health visiting in the council house, as it were — which I contend is the cause of much of the disaffection between these two groups of nurses who have so much in common and whose very survival may depend on their close collegial co-operation. I may be laying myself open to an indictment of negligence in not having written the appropriate chapter myself, but my ahistorical past made me reticent to take on such a task. Nevertheless, it is the understanding of the differences in development of district nursing and health visiting which have made the present situation comprehensible to me. In other words, the use of history has helped me to unravel a situation which I could not otherwise have hoped to understand. At the least, it has helped me to be more tolerant in sometimes exasperating circumstances but, at best, a recognition of our different pasts can be used as a basis on which to build future strategies for joint endeavours, if that is what we want. I can only hope, then, that an authentic account of this particular aspect of nursing history is not too far away.[1]

However, an example of how to use history is certainly provided by Celia Davies's chapter on nurse education. When Davies first planned her research into this field she was warned that it would be a waste of time to try to compare the development of nursing in Britain and the United States of America — they were so different as not to lend themselves to any meaningful comparison. She has shown that the very differences in approach to educating nurses, originating in the first place from almost identical premises, help us to make sense of the here and now. They demonstrate how, in different ways, both American and British nursing are economic and social casualties. New institutions, new structures to administer the nursing profession, will by themselves bring little change. A cake which is too small will remain too small even if cut in a different way, however ingenious that way may be. M. E. Newton, in an article making a case for historical research, reminds us of the famous warning: 'those individuals who cannot remember the past will be condemned to repeat it'.[2] Restructuring, without additional resources, will only condemn us to repeat our history yet again. To break out of our own past will require not only an historical awareness of having a problem but a recognition of forces, like the anti-feminism indicated by Versluysen, which are ranged against us, particularly when it comes to wanting more resources.

To the anti-feminism arraigned against nurses as a largely female profession (male recruitment is in any case said to be falling again) some would wish to add its anti-materialistic streak. Certainly Bellaby and Oribabor, using a method of historical materialism, would wish to count themselves among those wishing to break this down. Many nurses may find this particular chapter, with its frankly Marxist orientation, more difficult to accept than anything else in this book, but to me it poses a different but no less intriguing question. When does the present end and history begin? In the quotation which precedes their chapter, Bellaby and Oribabor indicate that to them the study of the past is only legitimate as a means of writing the history of the present. In a way, that is what I have tried to argue myself, but on the whole I think that I have argued for using the past to explain the present and predict the future. To base one's analysis of the present and one's prediction of the future on an investigation which will be little more than two years old when this book will be generally available may to some readers appear foolhardy. Yet one cannot but admire the authors for exposing themselves to the one danger which the general public normally expects historians to avoid, that of being proved wrong. It may well be possible for future readers not so much to say 'I don't agree with that' as to say 'events have proved them wrong'.

If this is so, then readers will have arrived at a moment of certainty, one of the few this book will offer them. Most of the time they will be confronted by uncertainty, by being forced to doubt those very facts which they either accepted as unchallengeable or regarded as self-evident and thus not worth questioning. People generally like to have the comfort which being certain on a particular point generates, and nurses grounded in medical certainty have craved that kind of security more than most. Yet here is nursing, already challenged in its most cherished beliefs by the emergence of research into its clinical practice, having its historical beliefs also undermined by the emergence of historical research into nursing.

The similarities between clinical and historical research have forced themselves upon my consciousness again and again in reading this volume. The difficulties of identifying the problem, the importance of the method in clarifying it, are identical. Christopher Maggs's chapter illustrates this well. His endeavour is to compare the 'prescriptive' model of nursing from 1881 to 1921 with the reality as contained in the pages of nurses' registers and matrons' report books in four provincial hospitals: Manchester, Leeds, Southampton and Portsmouth. His findings as such are challenging and disturbing and demonstrate the difference between history based on an analysis of one type of documentation and that based on another kind of documentation. However, his discussion on the problem of periodisation is fascinating. How does one arrange and order material which spans forty years and what would have happened if he had divided his material into statistically regular periods, such as five-, ten- or even twenty-year periods instead of the periods mainly preferred by him as bearing historical importance, 1881–1913 and 1914–1921? What would have happened if he had classified material from interview and observational schedules into different categories from those on which he actually decided? An account of deliberations leading to decisions in more clinically based research reports to compare with the honesty of Christopher Maggs's report could well give additional interest to clinical reports.

A similar comparison could be made of the chapter by Foster and Sheppard. Again I was fascinated to note that access to the dead, the records and archives of nursing, requires as much know-how as access to the living, the nurses and their patients. Archives have no more been created for the use of historical nurse researchers than have clients or patients for the use of clinical nurse researchers. Both require to be treated with respect and consideration and access to either of them should no more be taken for granted than anything else in life – as this book has shown.

Nurses are demonstrating an increasing interest in their own history, partly because of their growing involvement in general education through the Diploma in Nursing and the requirements of the Open University. To date, they have too often been forced to make bricks without straw, to see their past mainly through the eyes of their founding fathers and mothers. Moreover, they have too often been forced to see their history as one of continuous progress instead of one beset by innumerable traps and pitfalls. This book alone cannot hope to fill the large gaps which exist in our knowledge, but it can make a beginning. Hopefully, it will cause more nurses to ask questions about their own past and encourage some of them to search for answers.

Notes

1. The best historical source on the development of the district nursing service is still Mary Stocks, *A Hundred Years of District Nursing* (Allen and Unwin, London, 1960). G. Owen, *Health Visiting* (Bailliere Tindall, London, 1978), gives an outline account of the development of health visiting, and some of the developments referred to here are also discussed in A. G. MacQueen, 'From Carbolic Powder to Social Counsel', *Nursing Times*, 58 (1962). Some recent developments in district nursing and health visiting are outlined in J. H. Barber and C. R. Kratz, *Towards Team Care* (Churchill Livingstone, Edinburgh, 1980).

2. M. E. Newton, 'The Case for Historical Research', *Nursing Research*, 14 (1965), p. 20.

NOTES ON CONTRIBUTORS

Paul Bellaby has lectured in sociology at Keele University since 1968. Previous publications include *The Sociology of Comprehensive Schooling* and papers on social control in the classroom and the organisation of social work.

Gail Bolton is a nurse and has studied sociology at the University of New South Wales. She has just completed a research project for the New South Wales Nurses' Registration Board on health visiting in Great Britain.

Mick Carpenter trained as a general nurse in the 1960s, and afterwards studied sociology at Preston Polytechnic and industrial relations at Warwick University. He is currently researching and writing the history of the Confederation of Health Service Employees.

Margaret Connor Versluysen is a nurse, sociologist and historian of medicine whose career began at St Bartholomew's Hospital, London, and includes nursing on the Continent and admission to the Belgian Roll of Registered Nurses. She has a sociology degree, has done postgraduate research at the LSE and Bedford College and has taught at the City University and at two London medical schools. The role of women in medical care is an important research interest and she is currently completing a doctorate on the historical development of sexual stratification of work in midwifery.

Celia Davies has taught in the fields of industrial sociology, the sociology of organisations and the sociology of medicine. She is now a senior research fellow at Warwick University. She is hoping to prepare a full-length book on her work on the history of nursing in Britain and the USA and is currently engaged in research on the history of child health services.

Mitchell Dean studied and taught sociology at the University of New South Wales. He is currently researching historical questions on the government and administration of poverty from sources in both England and Australia and is preparing a doctoral thesis.

222

Janet Foster holds the postgraduate Diploma in Archive Administration. She has worked as a professional archivist for six years and has been in her present post as District Archivist at St Bartholomew's Hospital since February 1978. She is responsible for the records of all the hospitals in the City and Hackney Health District and for those of the Bart's School of Nursing since its foundation in 1877.

Charlotte Kratz is a trained nurse, midwife, health visitor and district nurse. She has a first degree and a doctorate in sociology. Her particular interest has been in the care of the long-term sick in the community. She is currently editorial advisor to the *Nursing Times* and is a freelance journalist.

Christopher Maggs is a general trained nurse and a registered clinical tutor. He has a BA in Humanities and is now working on a PhD on rank-and-file nurses before 1921. He has been associated with the History of Nursing Group at the Rcn since it began in 1977. He is also working on a biographical study of Sir H. C. Burdett, hospital administrator and Fellow of the Royal Statistical Society.

Patrick Oribabor has recently been appointed lecturer in industrial relations at Ife University, Nigeria. His co-authorship of a chapter in this volume is based on research done for his PhD at Keele University. He is a registered mental nurse.

Julia Sheppard is a qualified historian who took the Diploma in Archive Administration at University College, London. She helped to set up the Contemporary Medical Archives Centre in 1979. This is a permanent Centre at the Wellcome Institute for the History of Medicine, concerned with the preservation of twentieth-century medical archives and records.

Katherine Williams is a graduate of Girton College, Cambridge, and works as an independent scholar. She is a trained nurse, holding a Midwives' and Health Visitors' Certificate and the Diploma in Nursing of the University of London. She is committed to the study of bedside nursing work through her care of the handicapped, elderly and terminally ill.

INDEX